DISCONTINUE LEECHES!!
AND OTHER STORIES
FROM AN ENT'S TRAINING

DISCONTINUE LEECHES!!
AND OTHER STORIES
FROM AN ENT'S TRAINING

AMIT PATEL, MD

Copyright © 2018 by Amit Patel, MD.

Library of Congress Control Number:		2018901028
ISBN:	Hardcover	978-1-5434-8037-5
	Softcover	978-1-5434-8036-8
	eBook	978-1-5434-8035-1

All rights reserved. No part of this book may be reproduced or transmitted in any form or by any means, electronic or mechanical, including photocopying, recording, or by any information storage and retrieval system, without permission in writing from the copyright owner.

Any people depicted in stock imagery provided by Thinkstock are models, and such images are being used for illustrative purposes only.
Certain stock imagery © Thinkstock.

Print information available on the last page.

Rev. date: 05/17/2018

To order additional copies of this book, contact:
Xlibris
1-888-795-4274
www.Xlibris.com
Orders@Xlibris.com
768319

Contents

Intern Year xiii

Second Year 44

Third Year 91

Fourth Year 124

Chief Year 165

Fellowship 204

Attending 264

To my family for all the support they've given to me, especially my mother, who was unable to see me complete my residency.

To my father, for being a family practice doctor in the boonies and whose stories far outnumber mine.

To my brother, who helped me develop my sense of humor.

To all the patients, hospital support staff, residents, fellows, and attendings I've met over my (short) career; obviously, this book would not be possible without them.

To Joanelle, who gave me the final push to start writing.

To Patrick, who was once so concerned about financial troubles of the House Ear Clinic, he wrote a letter to the hospital about my well-being.

To Becky, for much needed non-medical advice and a supremely objective eye.

And last, to the Bible, for helping me through countless weeknights and weekends both on and off call.

Disclaimer

All the stories contained within this book are true to the best of my recollection. I have gone to extreme lengths to protect the privacy of all individuals mentioned, especially with regards to patient privacy. As such, names, ages, places, times, and other identifying materials have been changed accordingly, while keeping the essence of each story the same. This book is not intended as a substitute for the medical advice of physicians. The reader should regularly consult a physician in matters relating to his/her health and particularly with respect to any symptoms that may require diagnosis or medical attention.

Introduction

People don't know really know what I do. They have a vague idea, maybe an inkling, a "kinda, sorta, can't quite put my finger on it" notion of what an ear, nose, and throat physician is, but by and large, they have no clue.

Or they know that all I do is take out earwax (or it's more official term, "cerumen") all day.

They cannot be blamed for their ignorance though. I myself had no clue walking into my first day of ENT rotation during my third year of medical school what the specialty I would soon join had in store. Partially, this is the fault of the specialty because we cannot quite decide what to call ourselves.

From most basic to most complicated:

Ear, Nose, and Throat physician

ENT (because it rolls off the tongue)

Head and Neck surgeon (probably the closest to reality, but we don't operate on the eyes or the cervical spine or the brain, so . . .)

Otolaryngologist (most common "fancy" term)

Otorhinolaryngologist (because the nose specialists don't want to be left out)

ORL (for the pompous who still want an abbreviation but disdain the common ENT)

With such a crisis of identity, how are others supposed to know what we do?

So what is an ENT? I suppose ENTs need some description nowadays, since they have become rare and shy of Other People, as they call us. "There is little or no magic about them, except the ordinary everyday sort which helps them to disappear quietly and quickly when large stupid folk like you and me come blundering along, making a noise like elephants which they can hear a mile off [because of their oversensitive hearing]. They dress in bright colors [as dictated by the scrubs issued by their hospital]; wear no shoes, because their feet grow natural leathery soles and thick warm brown hair like the stuff on their heads (which is curly); have long clever brown fingers, good-natured faces, and laugh deep fruity laughs [especially after fending off a silly consult]." Now you know enough to go on with.

If you've read this far, you will have (hopefully) realized that this entire passage has been copied nearly word for word from the introduction to J. R. R. Tolkien's *The Hobbit*. Most ENTs I know would appreciate this type of joke because, for better or worse, we tend to be highly nerdy individuals. Otolaryngology, in my humble opinion, is the nerdiest of all the surgical subspecialties, excepting perhaps the ophthalmologists with their extra *h* in their name and their notes that are written in code incomprehensible to anyone but themselves.

How did I get introduced to ENT?

I had been convinced throughout college and the first two years of medical school that I was going be an orthopedic surgeon. This was mostly because I didn't know any better and thought that plating broken bones back together and doing joint replacements was going to be the coolest thing ever. So when I received my schedule during my third-year clinical rotations and orthopedics was my first rotation, I felt like going into orthopedics was my destiny. Two weeks on a joint reconstruction service disabused me of this notion. Sure, you got to wear spacesuits when doing total hips and knees, but there was absolutely no finesse in the operation, just blood and bone dust, cracking and hammering, and moving along to the next one. Also, I simply did not get along on a personal level with the residents on service. This is not to say they were not fantastic doctors who cared deeply about their job, but I could not see myself in that world.

So what to do? Luckily, my next rotation was an elective surgical rotation. Unluckily, I had decided I wanted to try ophthalmology, but all the spots were taken. So I decided on ENT because, for me, it was close enough to the eyes. My only introduction to ENT (beyond a few lectures during my second year, which

I dimly remembered) was when I was an undergraduate working in a fruit fly lab. Among my many jobs, I was responsible for dissecting larval brains under a microscope using jeweler forceps. One day, one of the grad students walked by and commented that I would make a good ENT because, in her words, "they like doing shit like that."

So I ventured forth for a month with the otolaryngology service. And it was AWESOME. My first day on the ENT rotation consisted of an extended radical neck dissection, where I got to see for the first time all of the neck anatomy laid out in all its glory. It was (and still is) one of the most beautiful things I'd ever seen. It only got better from there. I saw the most minute of ear surgery, ear tubes, tonsils, thyroids, huge cancer operations, and base of skull operations done completely through the nose, among others. They used all sorts of scopes I'd never seen—lasers, debriders, strobes.

More importantly, I felt like I had found my people. My first day there, I awkwardly introduced myself to the head and neck surgery residents in the call room and found that I had wandered into a discussion about buying the new iPhone intermingled with a discussion of whether a new *Star Trek* series would ever have the same impact as the original in the 1960s. This obviously devolved into the age old question of which captain was better, Kirk or Spock. They were huge geeks, and I loved it. They seemed genuinely interested in making sure I saw all the good cases and took time out to teach me things. I had decided pretty much in one week that I wanted to do ENT, and I never found anything quite as interesting during the rest of my medical school training.

For those interested in what goes on during interviews during residencies, the above paragraph pretty much represents what I told interviewers.

But then.

Then.

Then.

Then.

Residency hit. Residency is like the Matrix. Unfortunately, no one can be told what it is; you have to experience it for yourself. Medical school may teach you the facts, but in my opinion, every medical student should have to rotate through the Department of Motor Vehicles for three months while getting four hours of sleep per night while a burly man named Theodore (but insists on being called Dr. Theodore), who smells vaguely like cheese and toaster strudel, constantly berates you for not knowing the inner workings of the government while asking you to buy him cigarettes and taking a shit directly on his or her head. Maybe then, as the medical students stare deep into the soulless abyssal eyes of this man Dr. Theodore, they may begin to have the inkling, the faintest idea, the slightest hint, of the dark, crushing, and sometimes pungent future that lies ahead; they may see in those dark eyes themselves but the worst version of themselves, a person devolved into a quivering shell by the procrustean nature of bureaucracy.

This may seem extreme, but it may be the only way to adequately prepare hapless medical students for the rigors of residency. Every resident has a dark moment when they consider quitting altogether. The medicine remains the same and interesting; it is everything else, the bureaucracy, the intimidation, the culture of "we have to break you down to build you up," the self-doubt, the insecurity, the lack of food, sleep, and hygiene, the loss of personal relationships, the crazy abusive patients, the death and morbidity and mortality, the condescension, the depressed feeling of "I spent four years in medical school and now have my arm in a man's rectum pulling out shit, which he won't appreciate," the hierarchy, the feeling that maybe you aren't changing anything, the misery, the drinking, the constant feeling of inadequacy, the imposter syndrome, that brings you down.

With all this, we must find a way to cope. We try to find friendships or at least people to commiserate with in our coresidents because at the time, they seem to be the only ones who realize what is going on, the only people to whom we can relate. The attending physicians seem way too far above and have somehow lost this ability, no matter how recently they finished their training. I coped by writing down stories of the interactions I would have on a regularly frequent basis with patients, hospital staff, and others, and through the wonders of social media, I could share them with my friends because it could not just be me who was having these experiences. To my great surprise, people (in medicine and not) responded favorably, and so I continued to write a story or two per week and more with time permitting.

This book is a collection of those experiences (edited for privacy of course), from my intern year in general surgical training, through my ENT residency, and into fellowship training and beyond. Medicine is and will continue to be an absurd field, and hopefully these stories will allow some insight into what doctors have to face every day.

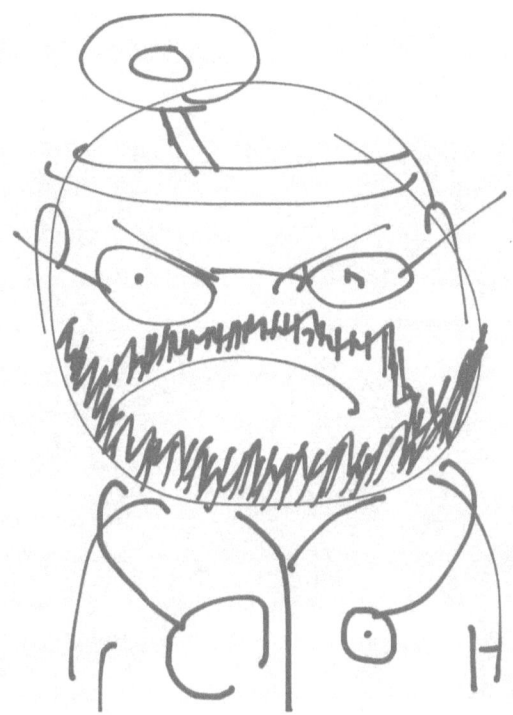

Intern Year

Why electronic orders should exist—Day 1 intern year

General Surgery resident: So this guy needs lower extremity duplexes. Do you know why?

Me: Cause we're planning on doing some sort of bypass graft?

Resident: Right. Do you know how to slip a vascular study?

Me: I assume there's some sort of form or order I have to put in. Sorry, it's my first day.

Resident: No worries, there's this form you have to fill out.

(*She leaves and brings back the ultrasound form.*)

Me: Oh, I see. You just fill out the indications and check off the study you want. Do I fax this down to Radiology or the Vascular Lab afterward?

Resident: Nope. Walk it down to the fourth floor and slip it under the door of the Vascular Lab.

Me: Um . . . under the door?

Resident: Exactly. That's what I mean by slipping. The Vascular Lab is closed right now.

Me: Yeah . . . so how do you know they actually get the order? You know, instead of just stepping on it or someone just throwing it out?

Resident: You're right. You have to make a note to call them in the morning, or better yet, go down there and make sure they know to do the study. (*She pauses and laughs at this moment seeing the perplexed look on my face.*) Yeah, I know it doesn't make sense. But this is the way it goes. Welcome to the hospital.

Me: Evidently.

Talking with my mom after my first day (and night) on call

Mom: So how did it go?

Me: OK, I guess. Still getting the hang of things.

Mom: That's OK.

Me: Yeah, definitely! At least none of my patients died.

Mom: That's good.

Me: And I didn't die.

Mom: Also good.

Me: And now I have a golden weekend!

Mom: Golden? What does that mean?

Me: Oh, it means I have two days off in a row. Saturday and Sunday.

Mom: So a normal weekend?

Me: Yes.

Plastic Surgery Grand Rounds

Attending 1: I'll tell you an interesting story. Once I drained a felon (abscess of the fingertip) on a farmer. Obviously, we cultured the pus that came out of it, and it grew back this very strange bacteria. I always wanted to write a case report about it.

(*Nobody seems very impressed.*)

Attending 1: Well, I wanted to write a case report about it because the same guy came back a few years later with a felon of the same fingertip. Sure enough, we drained it and cultured it, and it grew back the same strange bacteria!

(*Nobody seems very impressed.*)

Attending 1: Honestly, it's so interesting! I'm convinced there was a sequestrum of the bacteria that survived in his fingertip from the original infection that flared up years later. I wish we would have saved samples of it so we could run genetic analysis on the bacteria. I'm sure it would have been the same.

Attending 2: Well, I can tell you why he got the same infection.

Attending 1: Why?

Attending 2: Because he went back to the same shitty environment!

Attending 1: No, that can't be right.

Me, *leaning over to Plastics resident*: Is this how all of your grand rounds go?

Plastics resident: Pretty much. Just wait till you get to ENT. It's essentially the same thing, except you'll be arguing about the ear.

Me: Great! Looking forward to it.

At plastic surgery grand rounds. Again. One of the residents has just finished presenting a case.

Attending: You know, these complications are definitely a visual thing. Those pictures weren't that great.

Resident: Yeah, sorry, I took them with my phone.

Attending: You know, as plastic surgeons, you all should have a dedicated digital camera. The phone isn't good enough. Plus you shouldn't have pictures on your phone anyway, what with privacy rules.

Resident: OK.

Attending, *addressing group*: I mean, I don't know why all of you don't have a nice digital camera to take pictures of all these things. You can get a good one for like only three hundred to four hundred bucks!

(*Silence as the residents contemplate ever having that much spending money.*)

On call overnight

Senior resident: OK, you need to go see this fifteen-year-old kid and get him to eat.

Me: OK . . .

Senior: We admitted him for appendicitis, and he seems to be getting better on antibiotics. But he's still refusing to eat. If he eats, he can go home. So you have to convince him to eat.

Me: Great.

(*Go see the patient, examine him; belly is still a bit tender in the right lower quadrant but not rigid, etc.*)

Me: OK, so you seem to be getting better. But you haven't eaten anything. Why not?

Patient: I don't want to.

Me: OK, because it hurts you to eat?

Patient: I just don't want to.

Me: Yeah, but there has to be a reason for that. I mean, you haven't had anything to eat for nearly a day and a half. You must be hungry.

Patient: I'm hungry. But I don't want to eat the food here.

Me: Oh OK. Why not?

Patient: Because it's gross.

Me: So if you had better food, you'd eat it?

Patient: Yeah.

Me: You know, if you go home, you can eat anything you want.

Patient: I can go home?

Me: Only if you eat something.

Patient: OK, I'll eat something. I'll do it for two things.

Me: What two things?

Patient: I'll do it for two things of ice cream.

Me: You want ice cream?

Patient: Yeah! Chocolate.

Me: I think I can do that.

(*Go to chart, write order for ICE CREAM TO BEDSIDE STAT! A couple of hours later, I was writing discharge orders.*)

ASKED BY THE CHIEF TO GET CONSENT FROM AND MARK A PATIENT WITH SUPPURATIVE HIDRADENITIS (A PAINFUL CONDITION CAUSING PUS-FILLED LESIONS) OF THE BUTTOCKS. SPECIFIC INSTRUCTIONS WERE GIVEN TO MARK THE ONE AREA WHERE IT HURT THE PATIENT THE MOST.

Me, *to patient*: OK, sir, please point to where it hurts the most.

Patient: It hurts here. (*Uses his entire hand to grab his left buttock.*)

Me: No, no, just use one finger and point to the one spot where it hurts the absolute most.

Patient: Oh OK. It hurts here. (*Uses one finger to encircle a ten- to fifteen-centimeter hyperpigmented area on his left buttock.*)

Me: No. Just one spot. With one finger.

Patient: It hurts here though. (*Makes wild circles on his left buttock.*)

(*At a loss, I try valiantly for ten minutes to get the patient to just give me one small area to mark. In the end, turn to the med student who has been watching this sorry affair.*)

Me, *to med student*: All right. Just circle that pigmented area on his left buttock.

(*He does so, and we leave.*)

(*An hour later, I get a 911 page to the OR.*)

Discontinue Leeches!!
And Other Stories from an ENT's Training

Third-year resident: Dude, what the fuck did you do?

Me: What do you mean?

Third-year resident: What is this area you marked? Where are we supposed to start? The attending wants to cancel the case! He wanted to have a tiny spot to start and you circled the entire ass!

Me: Listen, I tried so hard to get that guy to point to one area. That's what he came up with.

Third-year resident: That's fucked up. All right, we'll figure something out.

(*EPIC fail.*)

On my ER rotation as an intern. Have been growing a beard for a bit.

Me: Hello, sir, how can I help you?

Patient: YOU'RE NOT A DOCTOR, YOU'RE AN ARAB! EVERYBODY'S AGAINST ME!

(Arab *pronounced "A-rab."*)

Me: I am a doctor. And actually, I'm Indian, not Arab.

(*Patient lunges at me, is held back by restraints, seems close to injuring himself.*)

Me: OK, five and two for you!

(*Five and two being five milligrams of Haldol and two milligrams of Versed. The ER is the WORST.*)

Run into an ENT resident while on shift in the ER

Resident: Oh, hey, how's it going?

Me: Not bad! I actually am having a good night—well, good and bad.

Resident: How so?

Me: Well, they let me sew up a tongue, a lip, an eyebrow, and a forehead. And dodged three vaginal bleeders. Oh, and I did a perfect spinal tap! No red blood cells.

Resident: A champagne tap!

Me: Yup! But they're not buying me any champagne.

Resident: Too bad. They should. And you gotta dodge those vaginal bleeders. So what's the bad?

Me: Well, I had to sedate a lady who's three months into her pregnancy who refuses to stop using cocaine and heroin.

Resident: Whoa, that sucks!

Me: Yeah, I'm learning people can apparently be terrible.

Resident: Yeah. So you excited about ENT?

Me: Yeah, can't wait!

Resident, *grinning and shaking his head*: Oh man, just you wait. Just you wait!

(*What have I gotten myself into?*)

Comments when growing a beard as a resident

Favorite comments (in no particular order):

1. You're not a doctor, you're an Arab!

2. Are you a caveman?

3. What's up, mountain man?

4. I thought you were a new attending physician, I was thrown by the beard.

5. Excuse me, which way is Mecca? (x2)

6. Your beard is magnificently glorious! (Patient high on PCP.)

ON CALL FOR THE FIRST TIME AT THE VETERAN'S ADMINISTRATION HOSPITAL AS AN INTERN. ANSWER A PAGE AT 3 AM.

ER: Hey, we have a patient down here you need to admit.

Me: Um, OK, this is the surgical intern. What's the surgical issue?

ER: Oh, he doesn't need surgery. He just needs to be admitted to the hospital. It's a social admission.

Me: What? What is that?

ER: Oh, the patient just came in, and he doesn't have anywhere to go. So he's getting admitted to your service. Can you come and write orders?

Me: That doesn't make sense.

ER: Yeah, but you're up for social admission. Medicine was last night, Neurology the night before.

Me: This sounds made up. I'm gonna call my senior.

(Call the senior resident on call.)

Senior: Yeah, that's a thing, the social admission.

Me: So a vet can come here at any time and just get admitted?

Senior: Yup. And the services rotate. I know it doesn't make sense, but that's the way it is. In fact, sometimes when people are taking care of their old dad or something and want to go on vacation, they'll just drop them off here.

Me: What?

Senior: Yeah, that happened when I was an intern.

Me: Like dropping a dog off at a kennel? That's fucked up.

Senior: Kennel would be better than the VA.

Me: Wow.

HAVE TO GO SEE A CONSULT ON THE PSYCH FLOOR AT THE VA

Me, *to senior after seeing the consult*: Hey, that Psych floor is kinda nice!

Senior: Yeah, it is.

Me: I mean, ping-pong tables, flat-screen TVs. I think I saw a dude playing with a Nintendo Wii!

Senior: Granted, you have to have severe mental issues to go up there.

Me: Well, I've been here for a month, so just enough time for me to crack. One day you'll have to round on me up there.

Senior: Nope, you'll be on your own.

Me: Nuts.

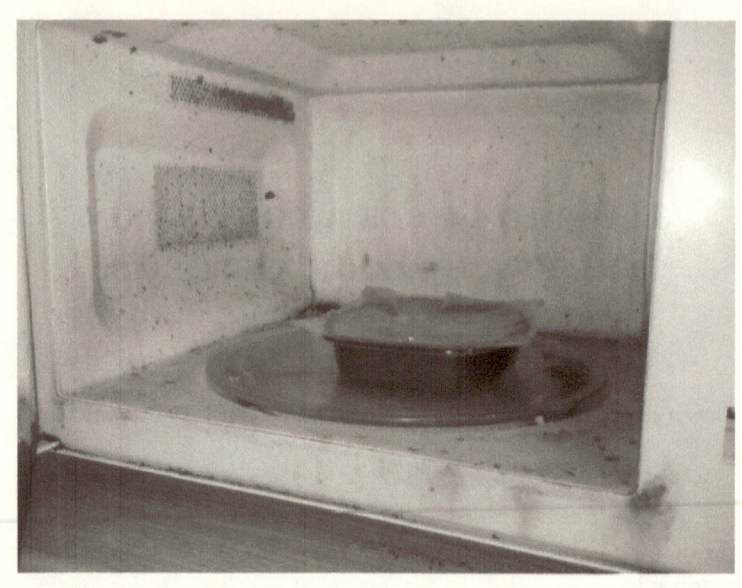

ON CALL AGAIN AT THE VA. FORTUNATELY, THE HOUSE STAFF GETS FROZEN MICROWAVE DINNERS BECAUSE THE CAFETERIA CLOSES AT 3 PM.

Senior: I'm going to order food. You want anything?

Me: I'm always hungry and can always eat. But I did eat one of those frozen dinner things.

Senior: You actually used that microwave?

Me: Yeah, didn't have much of a choice.

Senior: That thing is GROSS.

Me: Yes, it is. I tried not to touch any of the walls. Actually, I thought of taking a culture swab and seeing what grows, but then there'd be a mountain of paperwork that I'd have to fill out when it comes back as multidrug-resistant fungus or tuberculosis or whatever.

Senior: Oh man, that would be awesome!

Overheard in the ER

Patient 1: I'll break yo face open, NEGRO!

Patient 2: Don't call me a Negro, fool! I'm whiter than the crack you smoke! Don't you come after me now! I got 911 on speed dial!

(*Both of the gentlemen were white. I continued on my way.*)

GROANING AT COMPUTER WHILE FINISHING NOTES

Other intern: You look frustrated, what's up?

Me: I'm finding more and more, I answer the question "How do you, _____?" with "Do you mean at a real hospital or here at the VA?"

Other intern: Yeah, I know what you mean. This place is ridiculous.

Me: Yeah, I don't necessarily think a walking talking patient needs to be in the ICU, per se, but what do I know? I've only been doing this a few months.

Senior resident, *overhearing conversation*: Best not to think about it too hard. That's how you get cancer.

In vascular clinic at the VA, trying to get a patient admitted to the hospital for a below-knee amputation. Other leg has already been amputated below the knee.

Me, *to nurse*: OK, the attending wants to get Doppler studies of the lower extremities. I mean, I don't think he wants to revascularize anything, but I think he wants to document they've been done.

Nurse: Vascular tech won't do it because you didn't document that you tried an ABI.

(ABI = ankle-brachial index, ratio of blood pressure taken at the ankle to the blood pressure taken at the upper arm. Used as an indication for amount of blood flow to the leg.)

Me: I didn't do it because his foot is black. It's dead. I can tell you what it's going to be. It's going to be zero.

Nurse: They won't do it.

Me: But that's stupid.

(*Nurse shrugs.*)

Me: Ugh, fine.

(*Feeling silly, I put the blood pressure cuff around the patient's ankle.*)

Discontinue Leeches!!
And Other Stories from an ENT's Training

Patient, *looking down interested*: Whatcha doing there, doc? Chopping this thing off?

Me: Measuring the blood pressure in your ankle.

Patient: That's stupid. It's dead. Chop it off already!

Me: Oh, I agree.

Neurosurgery day 1. Senior resident is going through a CT angiogram of the carotid artery with a bunch of medical students who don't know any of the answers. I decide to join in and start nailing all the questions.

Senior, *at the end of the questions*: So you must be pretty interested in neurosurgery.

Me: Absolutely not.

Senior, *taken aback*: What, what? Who are you again?

Me: The ENT intern.

Senior: Oh, never mind then. (*Senior turns to the medical students.*) What the fuck is wrong with you guys? This motherfucker doesn't even care about neurosurgery, but he still knows all this shit. You guys need to read more.

(*Yet another benefit of being a resident—telling other people you really don't care.*)

Rounding with the Neurosurgery team. Patient has had evacuation of a subdural hematoma and seems to be getting better.

Chief resident: OK, so she looks good, seems to be responding a bit. Let's get a head CT.

Senior resident: She doesn't need a head CT.

Chief: But she's not vocalizing.

(*Junior residents and interns are watching closely because we're the ones who'll have to arrange for yet another head CT among all the other nonsense to be done.*)

Senior resident, *turns to juniors*: If you can get her to scream, she doesn't need a fucking head CT.

Chief: OK, whatever, we still have a lot of patients to go.

Working with the Neurosurgery intern and junior resident on call. Sit down after a rough night to go through everything.

Me: I'm fucking exhausted.

Junior resident: Yup.

Me: So much running around! Too many head CTs. Too many orders. Too many patients.

Junior resident: Yup.

Me: If my experience at this hospital has taught me nothing else, it's that we are all alone in this fucking world and you have to do everything yourself.

Junior resident: Yup. Welcome to being a resident.

Overhead in the ER while seeing a patient

Older white female: You're telling me my sister is the only white female in the Psych ward? That's unacceptable!

Harried patient care tech: Fuck you, you racist! If you don't like black people, stay the hell out of this hospital!

Morning neurosurgery rounds part 1: Chief is getting upset about the state of the list

Chief, *to intern*: Dude, what the fuck! We did surgery on this patient two days back. We took out the drain. How can there be not even a single lab? And now we just checked (*chief gestures toward the computer*), and there are labs present? What time were those labs from?

Junior resident: About two in the morning.

Chief, *exasperated with intern*: Two in the morning! What's going on here? The last labs you gave me for patient Smith who is the most critical patient are from 8 PM and there are three sets of labs after that! Here the labs are from two, and you're reporting in the morning that there are no labs present for this patient, and we look up the labs, and there are labs from 2 AM? Who's teaching you wrong? I need to put you on with residents who don't teach you the wrong method to follow! This is absolutely wrong reporting! You need to be on call with people who teach you the right way! The two most critical patients you have completely messed up the morning presentation! Completely! You don't have labs for either of them, and you said, "I don't know. There are no labs." For a person last night we were worried, we said she was herniating, sodium in the 131s. For the next patient who has a big-time EVD over there, you don't have any medications and you didn't know what the plan was. Third, the patient who two days past we did surgery, you said there are no labs while there are labs there! Who is teaching you wrong?? Not the way to do Neurosurgery. Not the way. Medicine maybe, not Neurosurgery.

(*Chief pauses for a moment and looks down at his list.*)

Chief: BAL, important event! Your ass should be on fire in the night! Like, "Holy shit, I hope I don't fuck up in the morning! Holy shit, I hope I don't mess up anything in the morning!" This is the patient we did surgery on two days back!

(Chief angrily looks at list and flips it over a couple of times.)

Chief: Next patient.

Morning neurosurgery rounds part 2: Chief cannot find a specific imaging result on patient and is getting upset

Chief, *to intern*: Either you put it wrong or you put it under another patient, and now we'll have to search every patient who's on the list, like where did you put the MRV on that patient?

Junior resident: It's listed under the image, but it doesn't auto-update into the comments.

Chief, *turning to midlevel resident*: These are things you gotta teach him! (*Chief then turns back to everyone else.*) And that is the one reason we don't allow PGY-1s to hold the call pager. Because despite a PGY-1 having a PGY-4 who's taking senior call, I have yet to reach a single patient (*chief holds up list for all to see*) who is pristine! That means just the way, not even hi-fi, just the way we present it every day. I've yet to find—I've gone through, one, two, three, four, five, six, seven, eight, nine, ten, eleven, twelve, thirteen, fourteen, fifteen, sixteen, and I've yet to find, please give me one patient in which I don't have to say, what the fuck! It's 6:15, I have three important cases! We've not had breakfast for three days now!

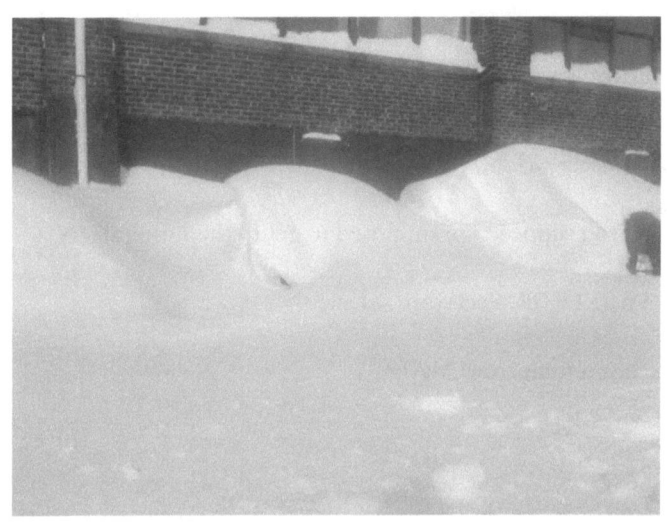

SNOWSTORM BURIES EVERYTHING. LOOK OUTSIDE, SEE THAT MY CAR AND PARKING LOT ARE UNDER A MASSIVE AMOUNT OF SNOW. DECIDE THAT I CAN'T GET TO THE HOSPITAL, SO I TEXT THE INTERN AND GO BACK TO SLEEP. GET A CALL FROM A MIDLEVEL RESIDENT LATER IN THE MORNING.

Resident: Hey, are you coming in?

Me: I can't. My car, the parking lot, the streets are buried.

Resident: You have to come in, we're dying here.

Me: I'd like to help, but I'm snowed in over here.

Resident: You have to come in.

Me: Hang on.

(*Send him the above picture.*)

Me: How do you suppose I'm supposed to get to the hospital?

Resident: Fuck. FUCK. Everything is awful.

Me: OK, see you tomorrow! Maybe!

New Year's Eve

Roommate: Hey, we're going out. Want to come?

Me: Nah, I can't. I gotta work tomorrow. Gotta be there at 4:30 AM in the morning to help round.

Roommate: Ugh, that sucks.

(*Show up at rounds the next morning, New Year's Eve, only to find the intern trying to sleep.*)

Me: What the fuck! I thought we were rounding at five. I was gonna help you preround and shit.

Intern: Nope, rescheduled to six. So I'm gonna try to maybe sleep 'cause it's kinda quiet.

(*Wait until 5:30 AM and then help the intern get the list together. Chief comes in to run the list. As we finish, chief turns to me.*)

Chief: So there's nothing to do today. None of the attendings scheduled any operations, so . . . thanks for coming in.

Me: What, that's it?

Chief: Yup. Who said you needed to come in?

Me: That's what they told me yesterday!

Chief: Whoops, oh well. Thanks for helping out, I guess.

Me: You're welcome.

First night on call as an ENT intern. Get a page from the floor regarding a Tylenol order.

Me: Yeah, that's fine, you can renew the Tylenol.

(*A couple of minutes later, get a page from the second-year resident.*)

Second-year resident: Everything OK?

Me: Yeah, just a Tylenol order. Nothing crazy.

Second-year resident: OK, just checking.

(*A couple of minutes later, get a page from the third-year resident.*)

Third-year resident: Hey, is everything good?

Me: Yeah, everything's good. Just Tylenol.

Third-year resident: Oh OK, good. You know you don't have to call me about those in the future.

Me: You called me though.

Third-year resident: Yeah, just wanted to make sure the pages were going through to you. Not that we don't trust you. But we don't trust you. Yet.

Me: Oh OK. Great.

Third-year resident: You'll be fine.

Seeing a patient for lip and tongue swelling in the ER with a senior resident

Me: OK, we have to take a look through your nose with a scope to see if this swelling extends down to your airway.

(*All of a sudden, we hear a commotion and huge crash from the bed next to us. The patient in that bed has ripped the monitor out of the wall and smashed it on the ground.*)

Our patient: Nope, I gotta get the hell outta here.

Senior resident: No, no we need to make sure you're OK.

(*In the meantime, the orderlies have gotten the patient in the next bed under control and dragged him off to a treatment area. All of a sudden, his family bursts in.*)

Other patient's father: Where's my son? I demand to see him!

Other patient's brother: Where the fuck is he?

(*They get progressively louder and angrier, and finally, an ER doctor comes up to them.*)

ER doctor: He started to get violent, so we had to get him out of here. And even when they do get him calmed down, the police have some questions for him. If you don't calm down, we're going to have security or the police escort you out.

(*Family continues to get angrier and angrier until the police come in and escort them out. The last thing I see before the doors close behind them is the patient's brother turn around and take a swing at one of the police officers. A few seconds later, the doors open, and I see the police beating the absolute shit out of this guy. Out of nowhere, another officer runs up and pepper sprays this guy right in the face. The doors close again.*)

Senior resident: This place is an absolute barnyard.

Our patient: Is it always like this?

Senior resident: Pretty bad today.

(Doors open again, and a patient near the door who apparently is in the ER for an asthma exacerbation inhales the pepper spray. While we're finishing writing up the consult, we watch as this patient is intubated.)

Me: Jeez, it really is bad today!

Senior resident: Yup.

Home call, 2 AM, VA paging

Me: Hi, it's ENT, what's going on?

Nurse: ENT? I have a consult for you. A patient here has a sore throat after an EGD.

(EGD = Esophagogastroduodenoscopy, or upper GI scope. Essentially a GI physician puts a scope through your mouth into your esophagus.)

Me: I don't understand. Is the patient about to die? And are you serious?

Nurse: Can you come in a write an order for ice chips?

Me: I'm hanging up the phone now.

In clinic, seeing a patient for nasal issues

Patient: My nose is really constipated.

Me: You mean congested. Your nose is congested.

Patient: No, man, I mean constipated. My nose is full of shit!

Me: Nice.

In the middle of a crazy day, seeing consults, doing floor work, etc. Get a page from the operating room in the midst of all this.

Me: It's ENT, what's up?

Anesthesiologist: We need you to come change a tracheostomy tube.

Me: What?

Anesthesiologist: This guy, he's having a urology procedure, and he has an uncuffed tube in. So we need you to come and change it to a cuffed one so we can give him anesthesia.

Me: I don't understand. Is it a new tracheostomy?

Anesthesiologist: No, he's had it for fifteen years.

Me: So just change it out yourself! You don't need me to come do it.

Anesthesiologist: What?

Me: Yeah, it's a stable stoma. Just change it. It's fine.

Anesthesiologist: No, you need to come and do it.

Me: No way, that's silly. But if you want me to do it, I have some urgent consults that I need to see first, so it'll be a while.

Anesthesiologist: I don't like your tone. I want to talk to your attending.

Me: All right, fine, go ahead. I have more important stuff to do.

(*A couple of hours later, the fourth-year resident finds me.*)

Resident: Dude, did you know you were yelling at the head of the Anesthesia Department?

Me: Nope.

Resident, *laughing*: Yeah, he wasn't happy. Came to find our chairman while he was operating.

Me: Oh shit, really?

Resident: Yeah, don't worry about it, our chairman couldn't believe it either. So you're good.

Me: Awesome.

Resident: And you're learning the annoying shit you have to deal with. It's good.

CALL FROM ER

Me: What's going on?

ER doc: This is one of the residents from the ER. I just saw a patient with quinsy (old name for peritonsillar abscess). I drained it, and I'm calling you to make a follow-up appointment.

Me: Holy crap, you drained a peritonsillar abscess? Usually, we have to go down and do all that ourselves.

ER doc: Well, it seems silly to call you for that.

Me: You'll make a fine ER doctor.

ER doc, *laughing*: Actually, I'm one of the Plastics interns just doing a rotation down here.

Me: So you were showing the ER residents what's what! I love it. Looking forward to working with you soon!

Plastics resident: Me too!

Working through a particularly painful clinic with a particularly painful attending. At this point, I've been on the ENT rotation for ten weeks and am exhausted.

Attending, *at the end of the clinic*: I need to talk to you.

Me: What's up?

Attending: How old are you?

Me: What?

Attending: You heard me. How old are you?

Me: I'm twenty-six years old.

Attending: How is it a twenty-six-year-old can't even string together two words to tell me what is going on with a patient?

Me: Um.

Attending: You have no idea what's going on half the time. You just sit there like a useless lump of a human being. And it's like pulling teeth to get you to say anything!

Me: Um.

Attending: Like now! You just sit there with this blank look on your face like you don't care. You are one of the worst residents I've ever worked with. I don't know

Discontinue Leeches!!
And Other Stories from an ENT's Training

if this (*attending waves hand around my face*) is just part of your whole shtick, but you have to fix it or we're going to have real problem. Now get out of my sight.

(*Go to the call room in a daze.*)

Second-year resident: Whoa, you look terrible.

Me: Just got destroyed in clinic by our attending.

Resident: You got yelled at?

Me: Yup.

(*I start to tell the story but get stopped.*)

Resident: Hang on, the other residents are just finishing up in the OR. Wait for them.

(*Other residents come eventually, and I relate the story.*)

Third-year resident: Ah, don't worry about it, it's all part of being a resident. That attending will end up liking you in the end.

Me: Really?

Fourth-year resident: Maybe, but if not, it doesn't matter. Now you're really part of the team.

Me: Awesome.

GET A TEXT FROM SENIOR RESIDENT

Senior, *via text*: Did you get paged about that apocalyptic pneumothorax last night?

Me: Apocalyptic?

Senior: LOL sorry, no idea why it autocorrected like that.

Me: No worries, was it really apocalyptic?

Senior: Nah, he lived.

Me: Too bad, would've made a good story.

Rounding in the recovery room

Co-intern: Hey, let the chief know where we are.

Me, *via text*: We're in the PACU.

Chief: Yay! I'm on the can.

Me: TMI . . .

Chief: Well, I had to respond.

Me, *to co-intern*: Well, seems like our chief is pooping.

Co-intern: Must be nice to have time to yourself.

Me: Can't wait until I'm chief.

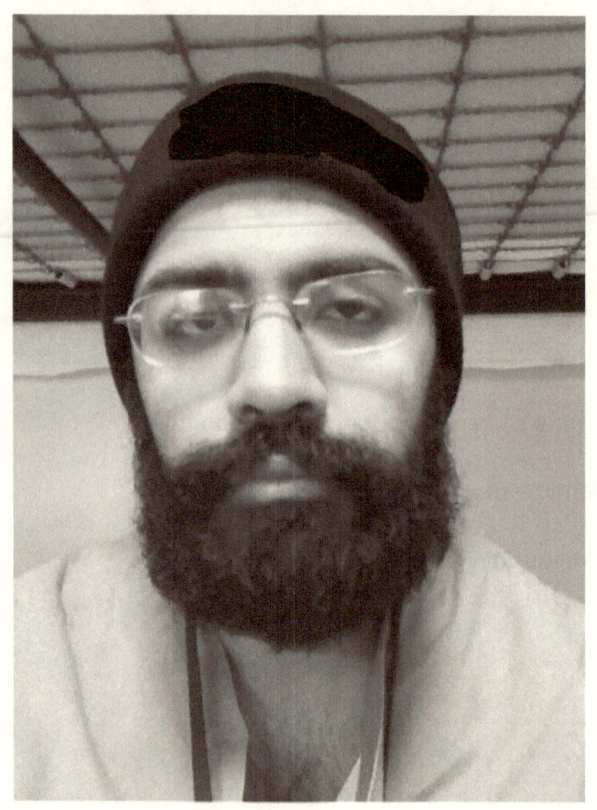

Second Year

Starting my first day as a PGY-2, a.k.a. the lowest person on the ENT totem pole

Chief: OK, so this lady stayed here last night cause the case finished late and our attending has a soft heart and let her stay the night. You gotta discharge her.

Me: OK, got it.

(*Go and write discharge orders for the patient. Get a call about an hour later.*)

Me, *answering page*: What's up?

Nurse: This patient doesn't have a ride home.

Me: What? Where's her family?

Nurse: We just talked to them. Her son's car got repossessed, and her husband is too drunk to come pick her up.

Me: What?

Nurse: You heard me.

Me: Um, can we give her cab fare or something?

Nurse: Let me put you on with the social worker.

Social worker: Yeah, we'll figure something out.

Me: Great.

(*Get called by attending.*)

Attending: Why is my patient still here?

Me: I'm working on it.

(*Get called back by social worker.*)

Social worker: OK, we got her a ticket on the train.

Me: Perfect.

(*Get called back twenty minutes later, in the midst of seeing another consult.*)

Nurse: We need an order saying it's OK for her to go home with the drain.

Me: OK, gimme like twenty minutes and I'll be up there to take care of that.

(*Finish the consult and then sprint upstairs to see attending walking away from the floor.*)

Me: Oh, hey, I was just about to discharge your patient.

Attending: Well, I just don't understand why this wasn't done earlier. So I took out the drain and discharged the patient myself.

Me, *taken aback*: You discharged her?

(As a rule, no attending knows the inner working of the hospital, much less how to actually discharge a patient.)

Attending: Yes, I discharged her.

Me: Oh wow, thanks. I'm just gonna go check on another patient on the floor.

(*Sprint to the nurse's station to find them laughing. Attending has written in the orders: "Discharge patient," and nothing else.*)

Nurse: We were just about to page you.

Me: Yeah, I figured.

ON CALL FOR MIDFACE TRAUMA

ER doctor: Yeah, there's this paranoid schizophrenic guy down here that decided to cut a keloid scar off his ear. Can you come fix him?

Me: Ah, yes, the Van Gogh special.

ER Doctor: Who?

Me: Never mind. I'll be down.

Getting annoyed by my pager

Me: FUCK THIS FUCKING PIECE OF SHIT! I HATE EVERYTHING ABOUT THIS PAGER.

Third-year resident: Two weeks in and you're losing it? That's about right.

Me: This pager is killing me.

Resident: My views on pagers are this. Your pager is an asshole. It makes terrible noises, the only thing that comes out of it is shit, and people are disgusted when they see it.

Me: I like that.

Resident: It's the truth.

Updating Attending on his Patient

Me: Plastics says Mr. Smith's oral free flap looks pretty dusky, so they want to start leech therapy.

Attending: OK, that's fine. Just make sure you tell the family before they start. Otherwise, they'll walk in and see all these leeches hanging out of his mouth and be like, "What are you doing to Daddy?!"

Me: OK.

(*Attending hangs up, laughing at the joke he's made. A couple of days later, I run into the Plastics resident.*)

Me: Hey, that flap isn't looking great. What's your plan?

Plastics resident: Flap is dead. It's going in the garbage, and we're going to do a pedicled flap instead.

Me: Awesome.

(*I head off to clinic and run into the General Surgery resident who is on her ICU rotation.*)

Resident: Oh, hey, what's the deal with Mr. Smith? I'm getting sick of getting these bait buckets filled with leeches from the Pharmacy. It's gross.

Me: Just talked to Plastics. They said the flap is dead, so I'm guessing you can discontinue the leeches.

Resident: Thank GOD.

(*Rounding in the ICU with the team later that afternoon and see the picture from the cover of this book.*)

Senior resident: Looks like they were excited to get rid of those leeches!

Me: No doubt about that.

SIGNED OFF OF A PATIENT WHO WAS ADMITTED TO THE MEDICINE TEAM AFTER WE'D DRAINED AN ABSCESS.

Resident: Um, the daughter of your patient is here and has some questions about the antibiotics you're discharging her father on.

Me: OK...

Resident: The daughter says she's allergic to penicillin.

Me: So what?

Resident: She wants to know if it's safe to give her father Augmentin, which is penicillin antibiotic.

Me: Yeah, I know what Augmentin is. Is the patient allergic to penicillin?

Resident: Um, no.

Me: What the fuck is the question? I don't understand. Is the daughter going to take the antibiotics?

Resident: So it's OK to prescribe this, right?

Me: Are you a doctor?

Consult from the weekend that elicited the same response from everyone with whom I talked.

Me: There's a guy in the Trauma bay. A car fell on his face.

Everyone: Excuse me? What fell on his face?

Me: A car.

Everyone: Ummmmmm . . . OK.

Consults at a private hospital

PA/APN/other underling: Hey, there's a guy somewhere in the hospital with [insert vague inane diagnosis]. His name starts with [insert any letter].

Me: OK... anything else? Room number? Vitals? Workup?

PA/APN/other underling: Oh, I don't have that information. Can you come and see him?

Me: Sure, why not?

Consult from Medical ICU

MICU: We have a guy up here that needs a tracheostomy.

Me: OK . . . He's medically stable to have it done?

MICU: Oh yeah, he's fine, we just can't extubate him.

(*I go and examine the guy and find that he has fixed, dilated pupils and no brainstem reflexes.*)

Me: So he's fine for the procedure? Medically optimized? You're hoping to get him off the ventilator after the tracheostomy?

MICU: Of course.

Me: I'm only asking because he's dead.

MICU: What?!

Me: Yeah, check into that and call me if he really needs a trach.

Finishing seeing an epistaxis consult in the ER

ER resident: Hey, I know you're here for another patient, but can you look at this lady with this neck mass?

Me: OK.

(*I walk over to the patient.*)

Me: Hi, I'm one of the ENT doctors. They wanted me to take a look at your neck.

(*Patient looks at me and immediately has a generalized tonic/clonic seizure, becomes stridulous, or upper airway obstruction, and her oxygen saturation drops to 40.*)

Me: Fuck. (*Yell over my shoulder.*) I'm gonna need some help here!

(*ER attending and resident come over.*)

ER attending: What did you do?

Me: Introduced myself, and she had a seizure.

ER attending: Well, we need to intubate her. Start masking her, and we'll get the intubation stuff together.

(*ER resident and attending try to intubate her and are unable.*)

ER attending: Shit, let's call Anesthesia.

(*Anesthesia is paged and comes down and try to intubate her and are unable.*)

Anesthesia attending: Shit, this lady needs a cric.

(Cric, pronounced "crike," is an emergent surgical airway when a patient cannot be safely intubated. *Upon uttering this, a Trauma Surgery resident and attending magically appear at the bedside with Betadine prep.*)

Me, *to myself*: I really just want to go home. If this lady gets a cric, it's seriously going to ruin my day.

Me, *out loud*: Hey, guys, can I try to intubate her?

(*Everyone looks at me.*)

ER attending: Oh yeah, we forgot you were here. Sure, you're an ENT and an airway expert. Have at it.

(*I successfully intubate the patient.*)

Me: OK, I'm outta here.

(*Call my chief resident.*)

Chief resident: What's up?

Me: I packed a dude's nose for epistaxis and intubated another patient emergently.

Chief resident: WHAT?

Me: I'm going home. I've had it with today.

THE SADDEST MEAL EVER—A DARK NOVEMBER TALE. CONSULTED ON A FRIDAY AT 6:45 AM BY TRAUMA FOR A FACIAL LACERATION. TRAUMA CALL ENDS AT 7:00 AM.

Trauma: There's a guy down here that was thrown through his windshield with a huge facial laceration. We had to whip stitch it shut because it was bleeding so much.

Me, *groan*: You couldn't have waited fifteen minutes? All right, we'll take care of it.

(*The guy has a HUGE laceration extending across the face. I call my attending who wants to take it to the OR but only after he's done with his scheduled cases. The entire day goes by, and soon enough, it's 8 PM, and there's no OR staff available. Meanwhile, I've been destroyed by a number of consults and floor work and finally run into the midlevel resident.*)

Me: There's no OR staff anymore. What are we going to do about this laceration?

Midlevel resident: Well, he's intubated in the Surgical ICU now. Why don't we just close it there at the bedside?

Me: Well . . . as long as we can control the bleeding, we should be able to do it.

(*Midlevel resident gets the OR to wheel a cautery to the SICU, and we start. I open up the whip stitch, and it starts hemorrhaging uncontrollably and the patient starts thrashing about. After paralyzing the patient, we spend two hours controlling the bleeding and suturing. When we're done, it's 10:30 PM*)

Midlevel: Have you had anything to eat?

Me: Nope.

Midlevel: Just go to Burger King and get whatever they have. I'll take an orange soda.

(*Go down to Burger King.*)

Cashier: Um . . . we only have four chicken fries left and whatever is left at the bottom of the fry basket. Also, our soda machine is broken and everything is flat.

Me: Fuck it, just give it to me.

(*Go back to the call room and start eating in near complete darkness. Midlevel resident comes in.*)

Me: I saved you two pieces of chicken and some oily french fries. Here's your flat soda. Enjoy.

Page from the VA

Me: This is ENT, I was paged?

Nurse: Doctor, your patient is gone!

Me: What do you mean?

Nurse: He's gone! He's gone!

Me: I hope you don't mean he died.

Nurse: He's gone! He got out of bed and drove home!

Me: So what do you want me to do?

Nurse: You need to come here and write an order, discharge home against medical advice!

Me: What? Why would I write an order saying to leave against medical advice?

Nurse: But it's illegal! It's illegal! We need an order! You're coming now, OK?

Me: No. Absolutely not.

Page from Recovery

Nurse: Doctor, you need to come admit your patient.

Me: My patient? He's going home after six hours of observation.

Nurse: But you need to come admit him!

Me: I don't understand. I wrote all the transfer orders to the recovery unit.

Nurse: I know, but he's bored and wants to watch TV. Can you admit him to a room with a television?

Me: No. Absolutely not. He's going home in six hours! He can watch all the television he wants at home!

Nurse: But he's really bored!

Me: What planet do you live on? I'm not admitting someone so they can watch TV!

Nurse: So you're not coming?

FOR MUCH OF MY SECOND-YEAR ROTATION, I HAD A PRETTY HEAVY BEARD GOING (SEE INTRO TO THIS SECTION). THESE WERE MY FAVORITE COMMENTS.

Favorite beard comments (in no particular order)

1. How's it going, Ted?

2. How's that cabin in Montana working out?

3. As-Salamu Alaykum, doctor!

4. Are you feeling all right? You're not depressed, are you?

5. That beard is fierce!

6. I'm too Asian to grow a beard like that.

7. Are you Gujarati? Then why do you have that beard?

8. Hey! It's Lumberjack Patel!

9. Are you Santa Claus?

10. Do you direct your own life, or does your beard take care of that for you?

Call from the ER

ER PA: There's this lady down here with really bad left ear pain and was told a year ago that she has a hole in her eardrum and that she needs surgery. Can you come admit her?

Me: What? Does she have drainage? An infection? Hearing loss? Anything?

ER PA: No. But she did have jaw surgery on the left side for a dislocated temporomandibular joint and was told a hole in eardrum is a complication.

Me: That's ridiculous. Are you sure it's not jaw pain causing the ear pain?

ER PA: Can you just come and look?

Me: Fine. But I'm telling you this consult is garbage.

ER PA: But you haven't even seen the patient!

Me: I'm just telling you based on experience.

Page from the VA

Me: This is ENT, I was paged?

Nurse: Hi, doctor, you have patient Smith?

Me: No . . . we don't have anyone admitted to the ENT service.

Nurse: It's the patient with the cataract surgery.

Me: That's the eyes. This is ENT.

Nurse: So you don't have this patient?

Me: This is Ears, Nose, and Throat. Not eyes.

Nurse: Really? Since when?

Me: I don't know. Since at least the late '70s.

Nurse: Really?

Me: Really.

Paged to the ER

ER doctor: We have a consult for you. It's for unremitting nasal pain.

Me: Really? Nasal pain?

ER doctor: Yeah, we can't figure this out.

Me: OK, I'll come see it.

(*Head down to the ER.*)

Me, *to patient*: Hello, sir, how long has your nose been hurting?

Patient: About three days.

Me: What happened three days ago?

Patient: Someone punched me in the nose.

Me: Great.

Me, *to ER doctor*: I'm done with you. Don't ever call me again.

Talking to an intubated patient's sister

Me: So they've called us to do a tracheostomy on your brother. It's a surgical airway inserted directly into the neck so they can take the breathing tube out of his mouth.

Patient's sister: Will it hurt him?

Me: It's a comfort care measure. They can lighten the sedation, and it assists in clearing his lungs and potentially getting him off the ventilator.

(*Proceed to go through all the risks and benefits of the tracheostomy.*)

Patient's sister: Well, what do you think I should do? Like if it were your family member?

Me: It doesn't matter what I would do. My family's personal wishes are their own, and my medical decisions are informed by my own life experiences. All that matters is what you think your brother would want.

Patient's sister: Thank you for being honest with me.

Me: No problem. Other questions I can answer for you?

Patient's sister: No, not at the moment. I need to talk this over with the rest of my family. Is that OK?

Me: Sure, take as long as you need.

Patient's sister: You've been so nice in explaining everything to me. Most people just want to get in and out. You've really taken so much longer than everyone else.

Me: Sure, but they probably are very busy.

(*Patient's sister thanks me again and then hugs me. Sometimes this is worth it.*)

In clinic again

Me: Sir, do you have any other medical problems?

Patient: Last year I called the ambulamps because I was bleeding from my butthole.

Me: I'd call that a definite yes.

Finishing up work on the floors with an intern

Intern: So we had a pretty good day, right? We finished clinic at 3:30, and now we just have to round on our patients and we'll be out by five, right?

Me: You goddamn fool.

Intern: What did I do?

Me: You said it. It's over. Now we are fucked.

Intern: Why?

Me: You don't realize. The universe has a way of knowing when you're about to be happy. And now that you've jinxed us, it's all over.

Intern: Why are you so pessimistic?

Me: I'm not pessimistic. I'm just telling you the way it is.

(*Two minutes later, airway consult from the ER.*)

Me, *to intern*: And here we go. I hope you realize this is your fault.

Consult from Pediatrics

Me: Hi, this is ENT, I was paged?

Medical student: Um, this is the medical student on the Peds team. It's for choanal atresia. You know, when there's no opening from the nose into the throat?

Me, *holding it together*: I know what it is. What's the issue?

Med student: Oh, we have a two-year-old here that we want you to evaluate for it.

Me: OK. Why do you think the patient has choanal atresia?

Med student: Excuse me? What do you mean?

Me: Usually, these things are discovered at birth. How do you know this two-year-old has choanal atresia? Are you able to pass an NG tube through the nose?

Med student: Oh, I don't know. It's not actually my patient.

Me, *still holding it together*: All right, is there a resident up there I can talk to?

Med student: No, I'm the only one here.

Me, *stoicism crumbling*: So you're running the Peds service?

Med student, *flustered*: Um, I don't know.

Me, *patience at an end*: Why don't you just go ahead and tell your intern, resident, or attending to call me before I agree to see this consult? Because this sounds kind of ridiculous.

Med student: Really?

Me: Yes, really.

An unprecedented TWO consults from the Psych floor

Consult one

Psych resident: We have a patient here that had diabetes. Now he says his right ear hurts.

Me: Does it look like it's infected? Is it draining any pus?

Psych resident: Well, I'm just a psychiatrist.

Me: I realize that, and I'm not asking you to make a complete diagnosis. I'm asking if you looked at his ear and if you think it's infected.

Psych resident: I'm just a psychiatrist.

Me: You realize I'm not a walking otoscope, right?

Psych resident: What?

Me: Never mind.

Consult two

Psych resident: We have a ninety-three-year-old lady up here who's catatonic and demented. We think she might have hearing loss. Can you evaluate her for a hearing aid?

Me: Do you think that will help the catatonia? Does she communicate at all?

Psych resident: No, she doesn't even move.

Me: So what's a hearing aid going to do?

Psych resident: (*Silence.*)

Me: OK, call back when you figure it out.

In the Radiology reading room waiting for Radiology resident to get off the phone with the ER

Radiology resident: There's a nondisplaced nasal bone fracture. The septum appears to be midline. (*Hangs up phone.*)

Me: Wait, what's the name of that patient?

Resident: Last name is Smith, but this isn't the patient you asked me about.

Me: I realize that, but you just said that this patient has a nasal bone fracture.

Resident, *confused*: Right . . .

Me: So any minute now the ER is going to be calling me about this guy. Are there any other fractures?

Resident: Um . . . I didn't see any other fractures. (*Starts scrolling through the images.*)

(*As she's doing this, the ER pages me.*)

ER resident: Hey, we have a trauma patient here—

Me, *cutting him off*: Last name Smith? Nondisplaced nasal bone fracture?

(*Radiology resident looks at me in amazement.*)

ER resident: Yeah, how did you know?

Me, *answering both him and the Radiology resident*: I live and breathe, my friend. I live and breathe.

GET CONSULTED FOR A TWELVE-YEAR-OLD KID WITH ORBITAL CELLULITIS FROM SINUSITIS, SOMEWHAT OF AN URGENT SURGICAL SITUATION. CALL THE ATTENDING ON CALL, WHO HAPPENS TO BE A DEDICATED SINUS SURGEON AND EXPLAIN THE SITUATION

Attending: Yeah, but did you talk with the pediatric attending? She should handle it. It's a twelve-year-old kid.

Me: Yeah, but I figured it's a sinus case, and you're on call and have operative time. Plus she's at another hospital.

Attending: Just run it by her and see if she wants to handle it. Don't want to step on any toes.

(*Hang up the phone and talk to the senior resident.*)

Resident: Yeah, our Peds attending got pretty annoyed the last time a kid came in with something like this and we didn't call her first. So just call her.

(*Spend the next three hours calling the attending's cell phone, calling the hospital operator to page her, etc. Finally get an irate phone callback.*)

Peds attending: What is the emergency?

(*I explain the situation.*)

Peds attending: Are you being deliberately stupid? There's a perfectly good sinus surgeon who happens to be on call. Have him handle it!

Discontinue Leeches!!
And Other Stories from an ENT's Training

Me: But he wanted me to call—

Peds attending: Good-bye.

(*Call the sinus attending, who starts laughing at me.*)

Sinus attending: OK, OK, get him ready for the OR.

(*Hang up the phone and turn to the same senior resident who happens to be in the room.*)

Me: I love looking like a jackass.

Resident: Eh, if you don't look like a jackass to at least one attending per day, you're probably doing something wrong.

Calling attendings to update them on their patients' progress. Get an urgent airway consult and run down to the ER to take care of it. About forty-five minutes later, get back to the call room and realize I didn't update the pediatrics attending, so I call.

Me: Hi, sorry about the late update, but—

Attending: I don't understand why you're calling me so late.

Me: I got paged to—

Attending: I don't care. You know, I do so many uninteresting cases over there, and you are always eager to update me on them. This patient from yesterday is the one interesting case that I really was interested in, and yet you fail to call me.

Me: OK, so—

Attending: No. Stop. I want you to listen to me carefully. The only thing you have going for you is that you're not Alejandro.

(Alejandro is the other resident in my year whom this attending also hates.)

Me: Uh . . .

Attending: Good-bye.

(*Third-year resident walks in about ten minutes later. I relate the story to him.*)

Resident, *laughing*: Wow, so she destroyed both of you with one sentence. Awesome.

Doing a nasal septum reconstruction

Me: How long do you want this bolster to stay in the nose for?

Attending: How long? I want it to stay on there until the guy can't fucking emotionally stand it anymore.

Me: So . . . like a week?

On the cancer floor to see a consult on a sweet old lady who's getting chemo

Patient, *as I'm finishing up talking to her*: Have you eaten anything today?

Me: Not really.

Patient: Because you look like you could use a solid meal. (*From a lady who looks like she weighs ninety pounds soaking wet.*)

Me: Actually, I'm going down the cafeteria right now.

(*I leave, thinking it's probably not a good thing when a chemo patient thinks you look like a walking skeleton.*)

(*On my way down to cafeteria, I'm paged by my attending's office.*)

Secretary: There's a consult. It's for hoarseness. They say it's pretty urgent, so you should see it now.

Me: Fine.

(*I go to the floor and find the resident.*)

Resident: Thanks for coming so quickly. This lady is really hoarse.

Me: Any medical issues?

Resident: She has really bad heart failure. You can't take her off the mask for more than ten seconds before her oxygen level drops.

Me: Well, that's going to be a problem if I have to stick a scope down her nose.

Discontinue Leeches!!
And Other Stories from an ENT's Training

Resident: Well . . . also she only speaks Russian.

Me: Ummmm . . . so how am I going to get her to follow my commands?

Resident: Oh yeah, she's also schizophrenic . . .

Me: Great. The trifecta.

(*I go to the room, only to find out that's she's been taken down to get a PICC line placed. I leave, with sandwiches on my mind.*)

Call from the floor as I'm eating lunch

Nurse: There's this patient up here you guys did a tracheostomy a few weeks ago. It fell out, but I don't know when.

Me: How's she doing?

Nurse: Oh, she's stable. You can finish what you're doing.

Me: OK. Just have everything ready when I get up there.

(*I finish my lunch in five minutes and go to floor. There's a crowd of people outside the room, like a code is going on.*)

Me: Shit. (*To nurse.*) What's going on?

Nurse: Oh, there's four respiratory techs in there. She's hypotensive and desaturating a bit.

Me: How long has this been going on?

Nurse: Well . . . since maybe ten minutes before I called you?

Me: But . . . I thought you said she was stable.

Nurse: She is!

Me: Doesn't sound like it if she's hypotensive and desatting . . .

(*I go in and see the patient. A bunch of the leads are hanging off, generating poor data, making it seem like she's crashing. In response to this, the respiratory techs are trying to bag and restrain a clearly awake, alert, and rightly confused patient who's trying to swat the Ambu bag away because she can't talk because of the hole in her neck.*)

Discontinue Leeches!!
And Other Stories from an ENT's Training

Me, *sigh*: Please stop. Please stop now. Please stop now. Please stop now.

(*I put tracheostomy tube back in and hook up the leads. Patient is "cured" and much happier.*)

Nurse: I guess I'll have to cancel the early response team.

Me: Another life saved!

Page from Peds ER, twenty minutes after I get sign out

Me: Hi, it's ENT.

ER resident: Hey, we just got the results of that CT of the neck you guys wanted on that seventeen-year-old. She has a four-centimeter abscess in her neck.

Me, *at a complete loss*: Who are you talking about?

ER resident: The girl who had the root canal last week that came in with swelling in her neck?

Me, *terrified, thinking that I had gotten a seriously flawed sign-out*: No one told me about this! How's her airway?

ER resident: Airway is fine. We consulted ENT earlier today, and you told us to get a CT of the neck. She needs to go to the OR.

Me, *perplexed*: You definitely consulted ENT?

ER resident: Yeah, you know, ENT or OMFS, you guys are the same thing, right?

Me, *righteously outraged*: No. No. No. No. No. Not the same thing. Not the same thing.

ER resident: Oh . . . sorry!

Me, *incredibly relieved*: Please, please, please don't call me about this again.

(One page, gamut of emotions.)

Page from ER

ER resident: Hey, we have this guy down here with cancer of the epiglottis. He's getting radiation therapy, and he's really hoarse. He's not in any respiratory distress.

Me: OK, I'll be in to see him.

(*I hang up the phone, but the patient's name sounds really familiar, so I look him up. Turns out he has active tuberculosis. I call the ER back.*)

Me: Um, you know this guy has TB, right?

ER resident: What? When?

(*He looks it up.*)

ER resident: FUCK. Fuck. I mean . . . what the fuck? Oh shit. What do we do? Fuck!

Me: Yeah. And I have to come scope the guy. See you in a bit!

(*I hang up the phone again.*)

Me, *to roommate*: Well, I'm gonna go get tuberculosis.

Roommate: Just take a shower afterward.

Me: You mean at the hospital? I'm not going to do that.

Roommate: Well, at least burn your clothes. I don't want that shit in here.

Page from Trauma on the Twenty-Seventh of the Month

Trauma: Hey, we have this patient down here that we need a consult on from ENT.

Me: OK...

Trauma: He fell off a ladder onto his face and has multiple fractures. (*He proceeds to list a bunch of facial fractures.*)

Me, *stopping him*: I'm going to have to interrupt you and tell you that we're not on for facial trauma today.

Trauma: But you're on the schedule for today...

Me: Mmmm... I'm on call the second, fifth, eighth, eleventh, fourteenth, seventeenth, twentieth, twenty-third, twenty-sixth, and twenty-ninth, for face trauma. So yesterday, I'd have been happy to help... but today you can call Plastics.

Trauma, *almost sounding disappointed*: Oh, sorry about that.

Me: No problem! See ya!

(Nothing better than dodging a disaster consult.)

Page from recovery at 11:30 PM

Me, *quite groggy*: Hi, it's ENT?

Nurse: Hey, doc, this patient here in recovery, you want him admitted?

Me: What patient?

Nurse: You know, the one who had surgery on his ear. He's having a lot of pain, so he should be admitted.

Me: Um . . . sure. Why are you calling? Please tell me you have admission orders.

Nurse: Yeah, he needs to be admitted.

Me: That's fine. Are you telling me that I need to come in and write orders to admit this patient?

Nurse: I just wanted to know if you wanted him to be admitted.

Me, *approaching from a different tack*: Do you have an order sheet with admission orders?

Nurse: Um . . . yes, I do.

Me: Then . . . admit him! Why are you calling me? You don't need to call me.

(*I promptly go back to sleep.*)

(*Another page from recovery at 12:15. Just enough time to get back into deep sleep.*)

Nurse: Hey, doc, the patient's wife wants to talk to you.

Me, *so tired I sound drunk*: Wha? What's she want?

Nurse: I don't know. (*Hands phone to wife.*)

Patient's wife: So he's admitted overnight?

Me: Yes . . .

Patient's wife: Well, can you get preauthorization for his hospital stay from the insurance company?

(*Ten- to fifteen-second pause while I try to comprehend what she's asking.*)

Me: What? I mean . . . huh? No. No. I mean . . . do you realize what time it is? It's 12:15 in the morning! What are you talking about?

Patient's wife: Hm. I guess we'll have to wait until tomorrow.

Me: Um . . . good-bye.

(*I hang up phone, wondering what planet I'm on.*)

Page from the floor at 1:30 AM.

Nurse: Hi, you know your patient who had the ear surgery? The one that had to stay overnight because the case got out late?

Me: Yes . . .

Nurse: She wants something to move her bowels.

Me: Ugh. I don't know. Any suggestions?

Nurse: We could do a lactulose enema.

Me, *silence for a good five seconds*: Are you crazy? I'm not giving a patient who came in for outpatient surgery an enema. How about some Dulcolax by mouth?

Nurse: Oh OK.

(Nurses love the enemas.)

Consult from ER

ER resident: We have a guy down here you need to scope.

Me: OK, what's the story?

ER resident: So this guy's neighbor was roasting a pig in his bathtub, and he set the apartment building on fire. This guy had a bad asthma attack from the smoke. We want to make sure his upper airway is OK.

Me: Wait, what? A pig?

ER resident: I'm not even making this up.

Me: Oh, I know. You can't make this stuff up. I'll be down.

(*Happy ending 1: I scoped the guy, and he's fine.*)

(*Happy ending 2: He and his clothes smelled so much like barbecued meat that it blocked out all the other smells of the ER.*)

Finishing up floor work and run into a fourth-year resident and chief resident. As we're discussing patients, get a call from a particularly awkward attending who want to round on his patients.

Me: Hey, you guys might want to get out of here before this attending shows up.

Chief: Nah, it's fine, we'll stick around and then make up some excuse to get out of rounding.

Me: Nice to be chief.

Fourth-year resident: Or just sucks to be the PGY-2.

(*At this point, we see the attending walking toward us with a couple of his own freshly washed white coats in plastic wrapping.*)

Attending, *to each one of us separately and with a slight nod of his head*: Hello. Hello. Hello.

Me: How's it going? You have one patient on this floor. We can start there.

Attending: Sounds good.

(*Attending starts glancing around as if he's looking for something. He then takes the white coats he's holding and tries to stuff them in between the white coat he's wearing and the left side of his belly and then the right side of his belly and then tries to button the coat around it. He decides this won't work and then stuffs both white coats into his pants and buttons the white coat around them. All of us watch this nonplussed.*)

Me: Um, do you want me to put those in my bag?

Attending, *noticing us watching him*: What?

Me: Your white coats. I can put them in my bag.

Attending: No way, these are valuable items!

(*The residents and I share a look.*)

Chief: OK, me and the fourth year gotta go to the OR. We'll see you later.

Me: Awesome, see you later.

Page from the floor

Nurse: Hi, there's a patient up here with a tracheostomy, and we think the trachea is coming out.

Me: Excuse me, what? What's coming out now?

Nurse: Yeah, you know, the cartilage rings of the trachea? We see a white ring under the tracheostomy. We think it's cartilage.

Me: OK, I'm pretty sure it's not, but I'll come and take a look.

(*I go examine patient and see a minuscule amount of white granulation tissue under the tracheostomy tube.*)

Nurse: Yeah, that white thing. That's the cartilage.

Me: Nope.

(*I take a piece of gauze and wipe the friable tissue away.*)

Me: See ya!

(*I run away, leaving a cartoon smoke shadow behind me.*)

Page from the Floor

Nurse: Hi is this ENT? For this patient Ms. Smith, did you guys remove her packing this morning?

Me: Yes, I did.

Nurse: Well, we were just checking up on her and we didn't see it, so that's why we called.

Me: Didn't you read my note from this morning? I wrote that I had taken the packing out.

Nurse: Well, I was just checking up on her for the first time today, and I didn't see the packing. I wanted to make sure she didn't swallow it.

Me: Did you ask her if she swallowed it? She's completely awake and with it.

Nurse: No . . .

Me: Regardless, I took the packing out.

Nurse: Um, OK. I'm just going to document that you took the packing out.

Me: But it's already documented. In my note. From four hours ago.

Nurse: Yeah, but just so I know.

Me: All right. Sounds good. I'm glad we cleared that up.

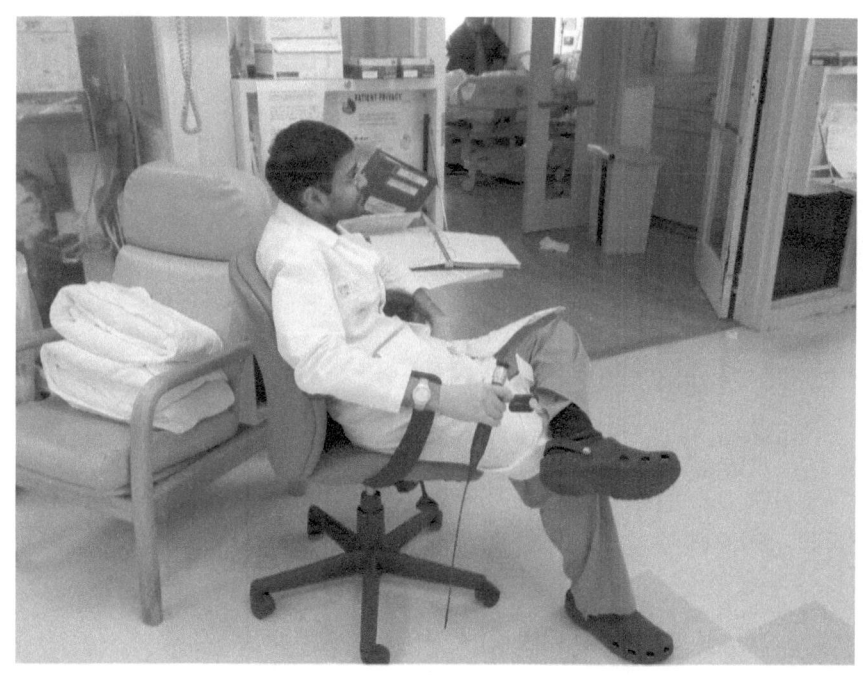

Third Year

4:30 PM AND AMAZINGLY WE ARE NEARLY DONE WITH ROUNDS

Chief: So are we done? Can I go home?

(*My pager goes off—PEDS ER!*)

Peds resident: There's a kid down here with a neck abscess.

Me, *groan*: Are you sure it's an abscess? Is there any way it could be an infected lymphangioma or lymphadenitis?

Peds resident: No, we're sure it's an abscess.

Me: All right. (*I get the rest of the information and hang up the phone.*) Damn it! Damn it! Damn it! Damn it!

Chief, *after each "Damn it!"*: Sh! Sh! Sh! Sh! Let's just go take care of this.

(*As we're walking to Peds ER, pager goes off again—FAST TRACK!*)

Me: Goddamn Fast Track! Goddamn it! Goddamn it! Goddamn it!

(Lesson to be learned here: NEVER let the universe know what you're thinking.)

In the OR, one hour into the case

Attending: This reconstruction we did before looks pretty good. I suppose we could revise it to see if we get a better outcome.

Me, *knowing that doing this reconstruction would be at least a four-hour comedy of errors/gong show*: You know, you always tell me that the enemy of good is better.

Attending, *puts down his instruments*: Huh, I guess I do say that. You're right. Let's stop here.

(The case ends. Victory is mine!)

Seeing one of our patients in the unit who has acute renal failure.

Me: So how's she doing?

Nurse: Better now. Her urine output has picked up.

(*I glance into the room, and the patient is talking to herself in tongues.*)

Me: Hm . . .

(*I go into the room. Patient is staring at the ceiling with her eyes wide open, babbling.*)

Me, *to patient*: Ms. Smith, can you tell me where you are?

Patient, *stops babbling*: Victory is mine! Victory is mine! Victory is mine!

Me, *to myself*: Fuck! Is she uremic? Septic? Altered?

(*I try four to five more times to get her to respond to me.*)

Patient: Victory is mine! Victory is mine! Victory is mine!

(*I put on a pair of gloves and perform a sternal rub. Patient screams.*)

Patient, *looks directly at me*: I'M FINE! I'M IN THE HOSPITAL! IT'S TUESDAY! STOP POKING ME! CAN'T SOMEBODY JUST PRAISE JESUS! VICTORY IS MINE! VICTORY IS MINE! VICTORY IS MINE!

(*I walk out of the room and speak to the nurse.*)

Me: She's fine. She's just having a Stewie Griffin moment.

Nurse: Who's Stewie Griffin?

CALLED TO ER TO SUTURE EAR LACERATION. WALK IN TO THE ER AND HEAR A MAN SCREAMING OVER EVERYONE ELSE.

Patient: DOCTAH! DOCTAAAAAAAAAAAAAAHHHHH! GIMME A SANDWICH! GIMME A SAAAAAANDWIIIICH! EVERYBODY ELSE GOT A SANDWICH! THE GOVERNMENTS GIVES PEOPLE SANDWICHES!

ER doctor: Sir, you need to calm down. If you don't calm down, they won't be able to fix your ear.

Me, *to no one in particular*: Oh god. Oh god. Of course. Of course, it's this guy. Of course, it is.

(*I go in to see patient.*)

Me: Sir, what happened?

Patient: My girlfriend hit me with a stick with a nail through it. GIMMEE A SANDWICH! MY GIRLFRIEND HAS SEX WITH EVERYONE!

Me: Uh . . .

Patient: MY WIFE HAS SEX WITH EVERYONE! I'M ONLY SUPPOSED TO HAVE SEX WITH MY GIRLFRIEEEEEEEND!

Me, *trying another tack*: Sir, do you have any other medical problems?

Patient: I GOT THE AIDS! THE AIDS!

Me: OK, you have HIV?

Patient: I DON'T GOT THE AIDS! I CLEARED THAT SHIT! GIMME A SANDWIIIIIIICH!

Me: Great.

Page from the VA

Nurse: Hi, it's Same Day Surgery, who is this?

Me: It's ENT.

Nurse: Oh, we were trying to get a hold of the day team. Are they still there?

Me: No. They left a long time ago.

Nurse: Do you have their pager numbers?

Me: Why? What's the issue?

Nurse: Oh, one of their patients they discharged earlier today came back here because she vomited at home. But she feels much better now.

Me: OK . . .

Nurse: Do you think she needs to be admitted?

Me: She feels better, though, now, right? Is she eating?

Nurse: Yes, she had something to eat before she came here.

Me: You mean, after she vomited?

Nurse: Um . . . yes.

Me: And she's fine now?

Nurse: Yes.

Me: So . . . why does she need to be admitted?

Nurse: I don't know. She's also asking for a copy of her certificate.

Me: What certificate? A medical certificate?

Nurse: Um . . . maybe? Do you do that?

Me: Nope.

Nurse: Oh. So you're not coming to admit this patient?

Me, *sigh*: No.

Page from Peds ER

ER attending: Hey, we have a kid for you guys to come and see.

Me: OK, what's up?

ER attending: There's this kid here. He's had a tracheostomy for the past four years, and mom says she left him by an open window yesterday and then saw a fly on the tracheostomy.

Me: OK . . .

ER attending: Anyway, she says she then saw maggots crawling out of the trach site.

Me, *at a loss*: Uh . . . maggots?

ER attending: Yeah. She thinks the fly laid eggs in the neck. Can you come and take a look?

Me: Are there maggots coming out of the neck?

ER attending: No, it looks fine.

Me: I don't understand. If it looks fine, why do I need to come and see it? You want me to look at a normal tracheostomy site?

ER attending: Well, the patient's pulmonologist sent him here to be evaluated by ENT.

Me: Did he see maggots?

ER attending: No.

Me: So both you and another doctor agree that there are no maggots. I mean... it's not dead and rotting tissue, right? You know maggots are only going to be around if that thing is completely dead. And you're telling me everything looks fine. So there can't be any maggots, right?

ER attending: I guess you're right. Can you come take a look anyway?

Me, *sigh*: I'll be in.

Page from the VA

Nurse, *talking extremely fast, hysterical*: Hey, doc, you know the patient Mr. Smith?

Me: Yes. What's the problem?

Nurse, *almost yelling*: You know, the one with the tracheostomy?

Me: Yes. What's going on?

Nurse: The one that had the surgery a few days ago?

Me: Yes! I know whom you're talking about! What is going on?

Nurse: He's on tube feeds! The tube feeds are at a rate of seventy! Seventy!

Me: Yeah. I—

Nurse, *interrupting*: But the IV fluids! The IV fluids are at seventy too!

Me: But what's—

Nurse: The tube feeds and the IV fluids are both at seventy! Seventy!

Me: What's the problem? Why are you calling me?

Nurse, *still yelling*: They're both at seventy!

Me: Calm down. Just calm down. What do you want me to do about this?

Nurse, *stops abruptly*: Are you in house? Can you come see the patient?

Me: Why do I need to come? Because his fluids are at seventy? I don't understand.

Nurse: I need an order to stop the fluids. Can you come?

Me, *long pause while I contemplate what has just occurred*: That's it? You need an order to stop the fluids? That's why you're calling? Just let the bag run out! And don't hang another one. And don't call me!

Nurse: But . . . I need an order.

On call day one of my ENT rotation intern year—called at 3:30 AM.

Trauma resident: Hey, we have a guy here that was shot in the mouth, and we think he has a pharyngeal injury.

Me, *to myself, freaking out*: Fuck. I have no idea what to do. (*To resident, after getting full story*) I need to call my senior resident. I don't know, we may have to come in and take him to the OR.

(*Make a frantic call to senior resident.*)

Me: There's this guy in the ER they just called me about. He was shot in the mouth. I don't know, I think we may have to go in and see him take him to the OR.

Senior resident: Is he intubated?

Me: Yeah.

Senior resident: OK, we'll see him in the morning.

Me: Oh, we don't have to see him now?

Senior resident: What would that accomplish? There's no real emergency here. He's got a stable airway, and we're gonna be there in a couple of hours anyway. Plus I'm sure there're other things wrong with him.

Me: Oh OK, but—

Senior: We're not seeing him right now. Go back to sleep.

(Try to go back to sleep, but nerves keep me up the rest of the night, or at least the one hour before my alarm goes off.)

(Fast-forward to last night—called at 3:30 AM.)

Trauma resident: Hey, we have a guy here that was shot twice in the face.

Me: Is he intubated? Is he bleeding? Do you have a maxillofacial CT?

Trauma resident: Yeah, he's intubated. He's not bleeding. We have a scan.

Me: All righty. We'll see him in the morning.

(I turn over and go back to sleep like a log. Seemingly, this is the new normal for me.)

Page from Recovery

Nurse: Hey, doc! You know your patient with tracheostomy?

Me: The one that just had a tracheostomy?

Nurse: Yeah! He says he can't breathe through his nose.

Me: Well . . . that's expected. He has a tracheostomy.

Nurse: Well, he says he can't breathe through his nose. Maybe it's blocked up?

Me: It's not though. The man is breathing through his neck. He can't breathe through his nose. It's physics.

Nurse: Well, can we give him some Afrin?

Me: Just because I'm an ENT resident doesn't mean that everyone gets Afrin. There has to be a reason.

Nurse: So what should we do about his blocked nose?

Me: Nothing! We do nothing!

In clinic, getting ready to scope a patient

Me: I'm going to spray some numbing medication in your nose.

Patient, *scared*: You mean with a needle?

Me: No, it's a spray. No needles.

Patient, *relieved*: Good, because I get PTSD about needles 'cause I was in 'Nam. And no offense, whenever I see an Oriental coming at me with a needle, I think, *Those bastards couldn't kill me with all their guns and bombs, but what the hell are they going to inject me with?*

Me: Right. (*I scope the patient, finish up the visit, and the patient leaves.*)

Attending: I bet you didn't know you were Vietnamese.

Me: That was news to me too.

SEEING A PATIENT WITH CHRONIC SINUSITIS

Patient: Doc, I feel so much better after that spray you gave me!

Me: I'm glad you're doing well.

Patient: But you don't know how excited I am! I'm like the cucumbers in that old joke!

Me: What?

Patient: You know, the one about the green tomatoes?

Me: Haven't heard that one.

Patient: So there's this woman who can't make her tomatoes turn red from green. She goes to the store where she bought them, and the guy tells her that at nighttime, she should take off all her clothes and dance naked up and down the tomato plants. The green tomatoes will turn red with embarrassment.

So she goes home and does exactly as the guy told her. The next day, she goes back to the store. "What happened?" the guy asks her. She says, "Well, the tomatoes didn't turn red, but all the cucumbers grew four inches!"

Me: . . .

Patient: See? I'm like the cucumbers!

Me: No, yeah, I got it.

VA CLINIC, SEEING A NINETY-YEAR-OLD GUY WITH A PAROTID MASS

Attending: So this doctor (*gesturing to me*) is going to set you up and do a biopsy on this mass.

Patient, *to my attending*: Thank you, doctor.

(*I go through the consent with him.*)

Me: Any questions?

Patient: No. *Gracias*, doctor.

Me, *to myself*: So this guy thinks I'm Latino.

(*I do the biopsy, all the while the guy is talking about how he was stationed in the Philippines and knew a lot of people from the Southwest.*)

Patient, *at the end of the procedure*: Hey! You're an attractive guy!

Me: Thanks?

Patient: It's a good thing I'm not gay! *Gracias*, doctor!

(Nothing quite like getting hit on by a ninety-year-old man.)

Consult from Fast Track

Nurse: This is Fast Track. I have a consult for you. We have this ninety-year-old lady down here that dropped a battery in her ear. I tried getting it out, but I can't seem to get it.

(Battery in ear = ENT emergency!)

Me: All right, I'll be there.

(*I drive to the hospital and find the patient. I look in her ears and see no battery, only abrasions and cuts in the left ear where the nurse had jabbed a pair of forceps into the ear canal grabbing for a phantom battery. I walk out to the front desk.*)

Me: WHO CALLED ME!

Nurse: I did.

Me. THERE'S NO BATTERY!

Nurse: Really? What was that gray pearly thing at the end of the canal?

Me: YOU MEAN THE EARDRUM?!

(*I proceeded to unleash a tirade of King Lear/Howard Beale/Les Grossman qualities, much of which is unprintable.*)

ROUNDING ON PATIENTS THIS MORNING WITH MY INTERN

Nurse: Thank God you're here. I can't take it anymore! She's crazy!

Me: This does not bode well. (*To patient*) How are you this morning, Ms. Smith?

Patient, *a cantankerous old woman starts taking and doesn't let me or my intern to get a word in edgewise*: I'm awful. My head hurts. Are these headaches going to go away? Why can't I eat my food? You took that tumor out of my head, but did you replace it with anything?

(*While she's talking, she's trying to eat a bowl of oatmeal and is fooling around with the packets on the tray, which include a sanitary napkin, Splenda, pepper, and jam.*)

Patient, *opening the sanitary napkin and trying to pour it into her oatmeal*: My daughter is a doctor, but she doesn't come to visit me. Are you boys good to your mothers? Why is there no sugar in this packet?

Me, *talking over her*: That's a sanitary napkin.

Patient, *still talking, picks up the pepper, opens it, and dumps it into her oatmeal*: My daughter's husband is a rabbi, but he doesn't pray for me. Are you boys married? Why is there pepper in my oatmeal? Why didn't you tell me that was pepper?

(*She fishes the pepper out of her oatmeal and throws it on her tray.*)

Patient, *still going, picks up the jam and opens it*: Are you sure your boss did a good job? I was going to go to Pittsburgh, but it was too far away. I couldn't sleep at all in the ICU, all those Spanish people up there. What is this red stuff in the packet? Oh, it doesn't matter.

(*She dumps the jam into her oatmeal.*)

Me, *pressing buttons on my pager*: Oh, there goes my pager. I gotta go. (*To intern*) Why don't you just finish up in here?

Call from my intern at 11 PM.

Intern: Hey, so I just got paged from this outside hospital. They have a patient in the ICU over there with a bad nosebleed. They say the guy's nose is packed, but he's still bleeding.

Me: Who packed his nose? Why don't they call that guy?

Intern: Well, they said that the doctor left a note saying if there were any more issues with bleeding from the nose, to call the ENT resident at our hospital.

Me, *long pause*: What? What did you just say?

Intern: Yeah, they said to call us. So I told them to hold pressure and put some Afrin in the nose. They want to transfer him here.

Me: No. No. No. No! Number one, we don't cover that hospital, so you can't be giving out recommendations for treatment. Second, who the fuck is this ENT doctor who packed his nose? He should get his lazy ass to the hospital and deal with this seeing as he saw the patient in the first place. Third, and this is for your own edification, when you're writing a consult, your entire assessment and plan is not allowed to be "If anything happens, call another hospital."

Pulled to the VA clinic

Me: What brings you into the ENT clinic today, sir?

Vet: I feel like shit doc! Forty-eight hours a day!

Me: Ummmm . . . so what's bothering you?

Vet: My feet! My knees! That other doctor says I got a circulation problem! (*Pulls up his pant legs*) See my knees (*pointing at his shins*), they all veiny and shit! They supposed to check that!

Me: OK, I'm sorry about your legs, but this is the ear, nose, and throat clinic, so what's bothering you with your ears, nose, or throat?

Vet: I ain't got nothing wrong with my nose! What you asking about my nose for? When are they checking my feet? That's what that other doc said! (*He pulls out a list of appointments.*)

Me, *looking at the list*: OK, it says here that you have a Vascular Lab appointment next week and then a podiatry appointment the same day. So next week is when they're checking out your legs.

Vet, *looks at me like I'm stupid*: I know that! That's what the other jellybean said! But when are they doing it today!

Me: We're not. (*I scroll through the computer.*) It says here that the last time you were here you were complaining of some dizziness? Like the room was spinning?

Vet, *again, looking at me like I'm stupid*: Doc, I ain't had that shit in six months! That shit ain't bothering me! What about my feet!

Me: Sir, this is the ears, nose, and throat clinic. Why did you come HERE today?

Vet: 'Cause they told me to! When they tell me to come, I come! I don't ask questions.

Me, *long pause*: All right, seeing as there's nothing with which you need my help, you're free to go. You don't have to come back.

Vet: So they're checking my knees now?

Me: (*Sigh.*)

Page from Fast Track at the private hospital at 5:45 PM.

Physician Assistant: So there's a patient here with a neck mass for a couple of weeks. We need you to come and see it.

Me: Um, why?

PA: Well, we consulted Infectious Disease, and they said to consult you for the neck mass.

Me: Well, tell me about the neck mass.

PA: It looks like a large lymph node. He's had it for a couple of weeks. It doesn't hurt. It's never happened to him before.

Me: Does this guy have an infection? Fever? Chills? Tonsillitis? Pharyngitis? Abscess? Skin lesion? Anything?

PA: Nope, just the neck mass. White count is normal. Infectious Disease wanted to consult you for a biopsy of the lymph node.

Me: It's nearly six in the evening. Send the guy home, and my attending will see him as an outpatient.

PA, *offended tone*: Well, just so you know, we're admitting him overnight because the Infectious Disease doctor isn't coming until tomorrow morning to see the guy. They wanted you to see it tonight.

Me: Did they now? Well, just so YOU know, we're not going to see this person tonight.

PA: Well, I'm going to talk with my attending about this. (*Hangs up.*)

115

(Call my attending.)

Attending: That's an absolute waste of resources. I agree. Even if that person is admitted, I don't want any resident seeing him. Just send him to my office.

(Always nice to get validated by your attending. Like getting a gold star on your spelling test in third grade.)

Highlights from a typical VA clinic

Patient 1: Where were you born?

Me: Buffalo, New York. But I know what you're asking. My family is originally from India.

Patient 1: I was born in Kazakhstan. I was an Israeli citizen. I'm a Jew. But I could never go to India. You know why? You know why?

Me: Why?

Patient 1: Too many cobras! You know what I'm talking about.

Me: I really don't.

(*A little while later, I'm seeing a patient with vertigo.*)

Me: Can you describe this feeling of dizziness a bit more?

Patient 2: Well, when it happens, there's all these flashing lights that appear in front of me. Then I get this feeling in my stomach and then this tingling that spreads all over my body. You know, like when you have an orgasm.

Me: Uh . . .

Page from private hospital

PA: We need you to come in and insert a NG (nasogastric) tube.

Me: What? I'm at home right now. And you don't need an ENT resident to insert an NG tube. Anyone can do that.

PA: Well, it's a patient that had cervical spine surgery and has a lot of swelling. He's in respiratory distress and needs to be reintubated.

Me: So what do you need an NG tube for? Just reintubate him!

PA: He has a lot of air in his stomach, and it needs to be decompressed.

Me: Are you joking? I'm pretty sure his difficulty breathing trumps that. Just reintubate him and stick the NG tube wherever you want.

PA: Um . . . so you're not coming?

Me: Not unless you're willing to wait thirty minutes for me to get there and put an NG tube into a dead person.

PA: Oh OK, never mind.

Page from the Floor at the VA

Nurse: Hey, doc, you know Mr. Smith?

Me: Yes . . .

Nurse: The patient that had the sinus surgery?

Me: Yes, I know who he is. What's the issue? I just discharged him.

Nurse: He's having hiccups.

(*Long pause.*)

Me: And?

Nurse: We're going to hold the discharge. You'll write the order? And you want to give him some medication?

Me, *incredulous*: Wait, what? Hold the discharge? What are you talking about?

Nurse: Yeah, he's having hiccups!

Me, *even more incredulous*: Can he not breathe? How bad are these hiccups?

Nurse: Well, he's having one every thirty seconds or so! You want to give him medication?

Me: Are you serious? No. No. No. No. No. NO! They're hiccups! Just let the poor guy go home!

Nurse: It's OK? I'm going to write a note.

Me: Do what you have to do. Just let that guy get the hell out of here.

Referral to the VA clinic for "clogged ears"

Me: What brings you to clinic today, sir?

Patient: Is your boss here? Can I talk to him?

Me: He's in the other room. Why don't you tell me why you're here?

Patient: My ears! It's a long story.

Me: OK. Why don't you get started?

Patient: Well, I saw my gastroenterologist yesterday. And he did that sigmoidoscope. And he wanted me to tell you about it. It's very important. I have it written down.

(*Rummages around his bag, pulls out a little slip of paper, and hands it to me.*)

(*The slip of paper says "DIAGNOSIS—ANAL FISSURES."*)

Me, *staring at paper for a long time*: What does this have to do with your ears?

Patient: Absolutely nothing! But it's something you should know.

Me: Noted.

(*And then the interview went downhill from there.*)

Patient walks into VA clinic

Me: Hello, sir, my name's Dr. Patel. It looks like you were referred up here for sinus problems?

Patient: You know, doc, you look real familiar. Are you a GI doctor?

Me: Nope, ENT.

Patient: I've definitely met you before. (*Pauses in thought.*)

Me: Well, let's check. (*Start scrolling through old notes.*)

Patient: I know what it was! You gave me a rectal exam three years ago.

(*I find the exact note describing said exam from my intern year.*)

Me: Um . . . yup. This is a bit awkward.

Patient: No, I remember! You did a good job.

Me: . . . Please tell me about your sinuses.

Page from Recovery

Nurse: Hey, doc, you know Mr. Smith? Interventional Radiology just did a biopsy on him.

Me: OK.

Nurse: He has a lot of pain. You write him for something?

Me: Why should I write anything? I didn't stick a needle into his neck. Call the radiologist!

Nurse: Doc, they're not allowed to write for pain medication. We usually call the person who ordered the test.

Me: You cannot be serious. Radiologists are doctors too! Why can't they write for it? That makes no sense. You know what? Never mind. I'll take care of it.

(*Sit down to log into my computer. As it's loading, page from Recovery.*)

Nurse: Hey, doc, did you order that pain medication?

Me: You need to calm down. We talked literally thirty seconds ago. My computer is loading.

(*I write for Percocet and morphine as needed for pain. Five minutes later, page from Recovery.*)

Nurse: Hey, doc, there's something wrong with your morphine order. Pharmacy flagged the order and they won't release it. They say you ordered it as a piggyback on his IV fluids. He's not on IV fluids. You want IV fluids?

Me: I don't want IV fluids. (*I look up the order, and it's ordered correctly but has been flagged.*) The order looks fine to me.

Nurse: You need to call Pharmacy.

(*Call up to the Pharmacy.*)

Me: Why did you flag my order for morphine?

Pharmacist: Um, it's ordered as a piggyback onto IV fluids and at a continuous rate, so you need to change it.

Me: The order's correct. I'm looking at it right now. There's no continuous rate, there's no piggyback, the man's not even on IV fluids! What the hell are you talking about?

Pharmacist: Hm . . . I guess you're right.

Me: Well, then, can you unflag the order so the man can get his pain medication?

Pharmacist: No, I can't do that. Once an order has been flagged, it can't be unflagged.

Me, *long pause*: Of course, you can't. Why would you be able to do that? I'm going to order this again, THE EXACT SAME WAY AS I DID BEFORE. You will dispense it. And you will not call me about this again.

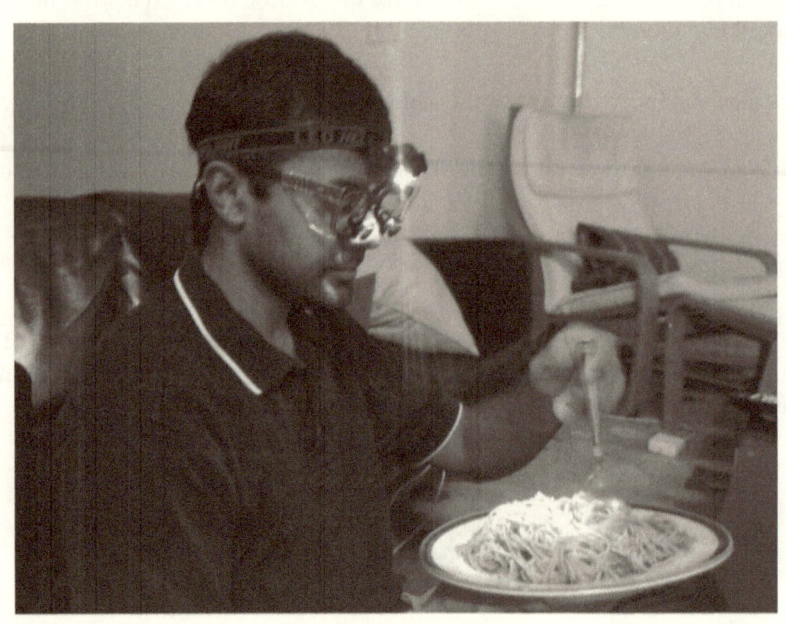

Fourth Year

Recovering from a bout of food poisoning from this weekend. Feel more or less OK when I woke up this morning, and have three cases to do. Cruising along more or less, until . . .

Me, *to medical student*: OK, just close the rest of this incision (approximately two centimeters) and we'll be done!

Medical student: OK. (*Begins suturing the incision in the endearingly slow way most medical students suture.*)

(*All of a sudden, I start to sweat uncontrollably, and my stomach begins to roil. Sensing something bad is going to happen but keeping it together.*)

Me: Um, why don't you let me finish suturing this together? That way, we can move on to the next case.

Medical student: Sure. (*Hands me the needle driver.*)

(*I throw the three sutures necessary to close the incision, put the needle and forceps back on the Mayo stand, turn well away from the patient, and vomit three times on the floor. The circulator sprints over and grabs the back of my neck to prevent me from falling out of my chair. All hell breaks loose.*)

(*My chief resident, who has been watching the sad spectacle, looks at the medical student.*)

Chief: Jesus, was your suturing really that bad?

(Needless to say, they let me take the rest of the day off.)

NEARING THE END OF A LONG CASE (APPROXIMATELY SEVEN HOURS). MY ROLE HAS BEEN MOSTLY TO OBSERVE, AND IN TOW IS A POOR THIRD-YEAR MEDICAL STUDENT WHOSE ONLY HOPE IS TO DO SOME SUTURING. TIME IS APPROXIMATELY 10:00 PM.

Attending, *finishing up the case*: So we're all done here. Amit, why don't you close this up? I'm going to go. Oh, and be sure to teach the medical student to suture. (*Attending leaves the room, followed by the medical student.*)

(*I start to close the incision. The medical student comes back in having scrubbed with his hands and arms dripping with water.*)

Me: Just get a gown and gloves on, and I'll have you throw some sutures.

Scrub tech: Dr. Patel, what are you doing?

Me: What do you mean?

Scrub tech: What are you talking about? I'm not sitting here while you let the medical student suture! It's ten at night! It's time to go home!

Me: But the poor guy's been sitting here all day!

Scrub tech: You have to think about others here. Anesthesia wants to go home. I want to go home. You want to go home. Med student wants to go home. I'll give him a gown as long as you don't let him suture.

Me: I can't promise that. If he scrubs in, he's going to suture.

Scrub tech: Then just finish up so we can leave.

Me, *to med student*: Sorry, dude.

Med student: No, it's fine. I understand. It was a really interesting case.

Me: No, it wasn't. I know you're just saying that.

Med student: Yeah, I am.

The following is a letter circulated to the hospital by a Neurosurgery resident with a particular sense of humor.

Colleagues,

The city of Los Angeles and indeed the entire west coast were shaken this week by the news of The House Research Institute's bankruptcy filing. For those unfamiliar with the Institute, currently bound, BNI-style, to the otherwise unremarkable (at best) St. Vincent's Medical Center community hospital: it is a veritable titan in the field of Otolaryngological Surgery. As in House Brackmann Scale for Facial Nerve Dysfunction you guys. It is a living, breathing Mt. Rushmore—a monument in and to the field. It is literally impossible to overstate the catastrophe of this bankruptcy, either in itself or as a harbinger of things to come (i.e. doom).

If Ear, Nose, and Throat Surgery is a coal mine, and there is a canary in the coal mine, and the coal mine was built under Mt. Rushmore, then earlier this week Mt. Rushmore crashed through the roof of the mine, killing the canary and most of the miners and destroying everything. If that makes sense. I'm not sure the extent to which the reverberations have impacted East Coast practitioners as yet, but my first thought, as was just now, I imagine, yours, was: What does this mean for Amit Patel, immaculately groomed ENT PGY-4 and Dept. of Neurosurgery favorite?

It's not good I can tell you that. Even if there is ENT in two years when he graduates, it will be the sort of medicine practiced in post-apocalyptic stories such as "Mad Max" or "12 Monkeys", and I don't need to point out that that is not, if you are a gentleman in the model of Dr. Patel, a milieu conducive to earning a living, much less building a new practice. As such, I've already begun taking steps to ensure that he will at the very least have access to shelter, food, and enough toiletries to groom in the manner to which we have all become accustomed. I've purchased a couch—which I plan on keeping for the foreseeable future—on which he may sleep at any time with little-to-no notice, as well as a stash of combs, fingernail clippers, and beard trimmers, that will at least support the bare essentials of his trademark groomsmanship. I've also sent him a personal check in the amount of forty dollars. I've done what I can. But remember I am 3000 miles away.

Please keep him in mind as you go about your day. If you find some change on the ground, think about leaving it anonymously in his white coat, hanging, pressed and unwrinkled, by the OR entrance. If you see him in the cafeteria, and you have some spare points, offer to pick up the tab on that bag of popcorn he likes so much. I'm not asking for car payments here. And remember that he is a man with pride and may not respond well to frank charity. But also remember that he is the one who provided us all with so much, including a video of me getting yelled at by a chief resident during my intern year, which has served as a touchstone if not the cornerstone of intern training ever since.

We can't—we mustn't—take him for granted. Otolaryngological Surgery may be collapsing, probably because they refused to see so many consults that people realized that the field was redundant and unnecessary, but I don't think any of us would be comfortable in a world where Dr. Patel is unable to make a living, destitute on the street with his shirt untucked.

Overheard in the OR: Anesthesia resident is walking about a four-year-old kid back to one of the rooms

Kid: But I'm thirsty!

Resident: Don't worry, once we're done, you'll be able to drink whatever you want!

Kid: But I'm thirsty now!

(*Kid turns around and sees an old filled suction canister sitting just inside one of the ORs. Fluid inside the suction canister looks remarkably like red Kool-Aid.*)

Kid: Kool-Aid! Kool-Aid! Kool-Aid! (*Nearly makes a break for it.*)

Resident, *redirecting the kid*: That isn't Kool-Aid! It's . . . (*Pauses for a moment and is clearly thinking if he should tell the kid it's basically a bottle of blood.*) It's . . . not something that would taste good.

Kid: But I want it!

Resident: Um, why don't we go into this room? There's lots of Kool-Aid in here.

CALLED TO TRAUMA BAY ON A WEEKEND TO EVALUATE A PATIENT FOR ROAD RASH OF THE FACE

Me, *to family*: We're going to have to take her to the OR to wash this out and close it up as best as possible.

Family: You're just an ENT doctor though. We want a plastic surgeon.

Me: OK, we'll give them a call.

(*Call Plastics resident and tell them the situation.*)

Plastics resident: We can see it, but we don't have anyone to staff it today, since we're not on call for Trauma and there is coverage for facial trauma. We can see it tomorrow if they want to wait. But I wouldn't recommend that.

Me: Well, I figured I'd give a shot.

(*Explain this to family.*)

Family: Why won't they come see her? All right, whatever you think is best.

(*A family member speaks up.*)

Family member: I work for a medical equipment company. Will you be putting her on heparin?

Me: Probably not immediately. That's up to the Trauma team who admitted her.

Family member: I understand. Will you be using the VersaJet to get down to the bone?

(VersaJet is a piece of equipment that shoots a razor-thin beam of sterile saline that is used to remove damaged tissue—a lightsaber made out of water.)

Me: Not particularly. We don't want be removing a lot of tissue from her face, and especially not down to bone.

Family member: Well, I think you should use it.

Me: Um . . . we'll keep it in mind.

Summary of a typical A. Patel call

1. Receive sign-out at approximately 6:30 PM on the way home.

2. Get called at 6:31 PM for airway consult. Turn car around and start driving to hospital. Mildly annoyed.

3. Called at 6:32 PM for foreign body consult. Curse the heavens.

4. Get stuck in rush-hour traffic and arrive at hospital at approximately 7:25 PM.

5. See consults, leave at 8:30 PM.

6. Arrive home at 9:00 PM.

7. Get called at 9:05 PM for bleeding after tonsillectomy. Resigned to destruction.

8. See kiddo at 9:35 PM with heavy oral bleeding. Calmly arrange for kiddo to go to OR.

9. Finally manage to get to OR at 11:30 PM.

10. Finish case at 12:30 AM.

11. Leave hospital at 1:00 AM.

12. Get called at 1:15 AM for patient who needs to be readmitted for postoperative nausea/vomiting. Wonder what I may have done in a past life to deserve this.

13. Run over some sort of animal at 1:45 AM on the highway going approximately sixty miles per hour and absolutely obliterate it. Consider this a perfect ending to my call.

14. Arrive home at 2:25 AM.

15. Paged approximately ten times between 2:30 AM and 4:30 AM for various issues.

16. Leave for work at 5:30 AM.

17. Arrive at work, pager off at 6:00 AM.

(ALWAYS a black cloud.)

PAGE FROM ATTENDING REGARDING A CONSULT

Attending: Hey, Amit, can we go round on this consult?

(Without going into specifics, patient is a crazy person.)

Me: Um . . . OK, I just have to stop by the call room. I'll meet you at the nurses' station on the floor, and we'll see the patient together.

Attending: OK.

(*Go up to the patient's floor and look for my attending. Hear a ruckus coming from our patient's room and I run in. Patient is nearly naked and is holding a Texas catheter [essentially a condom with a catheter attached to it] filled with urine and is trying to hand it to my attending.*)

Attending, *bewildered*: Sir, I just want to look at your face. Your face!

Patient, *brandishing catheter*: Take it! Take it!

Attending, *bewildered, turns to me*: Amit, can you help him with this?

Me: Not really. Sir, just put it down. PUT IT DOWN. We'll take care of that in a little bit, don't worry about that now.

(*We quickly finish our exam. As we're leaving, patient tries to give us the catheter again.*)

Me, *to attending*: I thought we were going to meet at the nurses' station!

Attending: That was unexpected. I'm never seeing a patient without the residents again.

Me: Probably a good idea.

Rounding on patients

Me: How are you feeling after surgery?

Patient: I feel great! Now I don't quite remember who you are.

Me: That's all right. My name is Dr. Patel. I work with the ENT service.

Patient: That's great! You work with the church of ENT? Can you get me a rosary?

Me: No, I'm a resident doctor. I helped with the surgery on your face.

Patient: Oh, you're the president? Can you get me a rosary?

Me: We're going to work on that. I'm glad you're feeling better.

Rounding on a patient who tried to hang himself

Me, *to junior resident*: All right, all we have to do here is make sure his voice sounds all right. If it is, we're signing off.

Junior: OK.

(*Go in to see the patient; voice sounds great.*)

Junior: Well, your voice sounds really good. We don't have any further concerns about your airway. But how are you doing otherwise?

Me, *to myself*: And here we go . . .

(*Patient launches into story of how he recently had two heart attacks, strokes, and how he didn't want to live his life anymore.*)

Junior: Well, I can see how that would be really tough on you. Just hang in there!

Me, *to myself*: NOOOOOOOOOOOO!

Patient: Well, that's what I tried to do.

(*Superawkward pause ensues. I leave the room to let my junior fix the mess he's now in.*)

Why words matter

Me: This is ENT, I was paged.

Nurse: We have a patient up here. He had inspiratory stridor.

(Inspiratory stridor = airway obstruction above the level of the vocal cords)

Me: Are you sure?

Nurse: Definitely. We called a rapid response on him three hours ago. We need you to come see him.

Me: OK . . . he had stridor starting three hours ago? Why are you calling me now?

Nurse: Well, he doesn't have it anymore. But we want to make sure he doesn't have a tumor or something.

Me, *realizing more pain will come with arguing*: I'll be there when I get a chance.

(*I start going through the notes. Various people describe the noise he was making as "nasal congestion" to "inspiratory stridor" to "expiratory stridor" [signifying possible obstruction in the trachea] to "wheezing" [signifying possible obstruction in the lungs] to "inspiratory stridor with quiet breathing" [which makes no sense].*)

(*According to these stellar notes, it seems like at some point, every part of his airway was blocked. Armed with this information, I go to see the patient.*)

Me: Hello, sir, I heard you had some difficulty breathing this morning.

Patient: Yup!

Me: Can you describe the sound?

Discontinue Leeches!!
And Other Stories from an ENT's Training

Patient: It was like a weaseling.

Me: . . . Um, weaseling? Do you mean whistling or wheezing?

Patient: My nose was weaseling! Weaseling!

Me: Perfect.

Why words matter 2: A story from medical school

Me: What brings you to the clinic today?

Patient: My arms are numb! All the time! Then I can't feel them! Then they go numb!

(*I try valiantly as any medical student would to get a more accurate history. The patient is having none of it and is fixated on her numbness. Puzzled but still eager [like any medical student], I return to the resident room to present to the attending. Attending is decidedly old school, having been practicing medicine since the introduction of penicillin.*)

Attending: Who has a patient to present? Anyone? Residents? Students?

Me: I have someone.

Attending: Let's hear it.

Me: This is a thirty-seven-year old female who presents with a chief complaint of numbness of her arms—

Attending, *interrupting*: Wait a second. Numbness? What do you mean by numbness?

Me: Well, she says—

Attending, *interrupting*: Numbness is not a symptom. In fact, if you ever tell me a patient has numbness again, I'll chop your balls off.

(*All residents stop typing, turn, and stare.*)

Me: Uh . . .

Attending: This is ridiculous. Numbness? I've never heard of that. If any of you ever use that word, I'll chop all of your balls off. All right, let's go see the patient.

(Moral: Use the right words or risk castration.)

FINDING COVERAGE, OR ATTENDING ROULETTE

Attending A: This patient was supposed to come to my office but went to the ER instead. Please see him and let me know if I need to do something.

(Patient turns out to have a large abscess requiring help from General Surgery colleagues. Call placed to attending A.)

Attending A: I'm operating at a surgery center today and I'm not available. Isn't attending B on call for the ER? Just call him and tell him that I can't make it and I would appreciate his help.

(Call placed to attending B. Explain situation.)

Attending B: Isn't this attending A's patient? Why should I be involved? Why is this my problem? Why didn't attending A call me directly if he wanted my help? I'm busy. Call him back and tell him I'm not available currently.

(Call placed to attending A. Explain situation.)

Attending A: OK. Actually, I called attending C just after you called. He's going to see the patient. I hope attending B wasn't annoyed.

Me: Well . . . hang on, I'm getting paged by attending C.

Attending C: Meet me in the patient's room in two minutes.

(Go to patient's room. Attending C is nowhere to be found. Paged again by attending C.)

Attending C: What room is the patient in? I actually don't know.

(See patient with attending C. Get paged by General Surgery.)

Discontinue Leeches!!
And Other Stories from an ENT's Training

General Surgery: We have a room available in half an hour. Which one of your attendings is covering?

Me: Attending C. He's seeing the patient right now.

(*Go back to patient's room and tell attending C that room will be ready shortly.*)

Attending C: But I thought this was going to go this afternoon. I have patients in my office to see. I'm not available. What about attending D? Isn't he operating today?

Me: Yes, he is. But I think he's got cases booked through the afternoon.

Attending C: Please ask him if he can cover it.

(*Find attending D in operating room and explain situation.*)

Attending D: Oh, I know all about it. Attending B called me to see if I could cover the case. I might be able to cover it.

(Call back attending C.)

Me: Attending D said he should be able to cover the case.

Attending C: Well, I just talked with attending B, who said that he's now available to cover the case.

Me: OK . . . (*Turn to attending D and tell him attending B is covering the case.*)

Attending D: Well, then, why didn't attending B call me in the first place if he could cover it the entire time?

Me: I don't know.

(*Paged by attending A.*)

Attending A: My next two patients cancelled, so I could pop over to the hospital and do this case if you can delay it for an hour or so.

Me: Apparently, attending B is covering the case now.

Attending A: I thought he wasn't available? What about attending C?

Me: He says he's not available. But I'm going to go consent the patient.

(*Consent for patient for procedure and put attendings A, B, C, and D's names on the form. Paged by General Surgery just as I'm about to page them.*)

General Surgery: Our attending was annoyed that attending A isn't covering the case. Right after we talked to you, he called attending B personally to have him cover the case. He didn't tell us.

Me: Perfect.

(*Paged by attending B.*)

Attending B: General Surgery is going to go first. I'm still in my office seeing patients. I talked to attending D, who might start our portion if I'm running late.

Me, *long pause*: All right.

(*Patient ends up going to OR with attending B. Post op, get phone calls from A, B, C, and D, all wanting updates on the patient. Want to blow my brains out.*)

Happen to fall in line walking beside a General Surgery resident. She's in the middle of making rounds with two medical students.

Resident: Hey, do you have any cases that we can cover? Say a thyroid here or there?

Me: Nothing coming up in the near future, but we'll always let you know.

(*At this point, one medical student turns to me.*)

Student, *EXTREMELY perky and holding out her hand*: Hi, my name's Kim! What's your name?

Me, *shaking hand, slightly confused*: Amit. Nice to meet you?

Student: Isn't surgery great? What type do you do?

Me: I'm an ENT resident.

Student: That's AMAZING. What are you doing now?

(*It was the end of the day, and I was trying to tie up loose ends around the hospital so I could leave.*)

Me: Just floating around the hospital.

Student: Oh, that's great. How long are you with us?

Me: I'm not with your team.

Student, *still excited but confused*: But you said you're the float resident. Aren't you rounding with us?

Me: I'm not a float resident. I just happened to be walking beside you.

Student, *crestfallen*: Oh. Well, it was good meeting you!

Me: Sure. It's been an experience.

(Med students are fun!)

Seeing a ninety-year-old World War II vet for facial swelling

Me: Have you had any surgeries in the past?

Vet: Well, I rode with the Free French Forces. Those guys rode hard! I had the worst case of hemorrhoids the army had ever seen. They had to call a specialist to operate.

Me: I'd say that's a big yes.

(*I quickly examine the patient, including a scope to check his vocal cords.*)

Patient: That went well! You have a very gentle nature.

Me: Well, that's kind of you to say. Thank you.

Patient: You know, I've always liked doctors. One of my roommates during training was the company medic.

(*He turns to his approximately sixty-five-year-old daughter.*)

Patient: Hey, cover your ears! Earmuffs! This story isn't for you! It's for my new doctor!

Me: Um . . .

Patient: He used to get us all the girls in town. Then he'd treat us for the clap afterward! And all the other ones!

Me: Sounds like a great guy . . .

Patient: He was the best!

(If you're a World War II vet and you've made it this long, you get to say whatever you want.)

Paged to the ICU

ICU: There's patient here with leukemia. His nose is bleeding . . . It's a slow steady ooze, and it's been going on for a while now. We need you to come pack it.

Me: OK, I'll be there.

(*Go to see the patient, who is in TERRIBLE shape. Pneumonia, on pressors, etc., but still able to put up a big fight to prevent me from packing his nose, while gagging on the large clot that's been slowly building up in the back of this throat. Apologizing profusely, even though I'm pretty sure he doesn't know what's happening, I manage to pack his nose and then spend good amount of time suctioning out his mouth to get the large clot from out of there.*)

Me, *to ICU resident*: So we'll keep that packing in for about three days, try to correct his platelets for what it's worth, and avoid anticoagulants if possible.

ICU resident: Sure thing.

(*Go through the list later and find that the patient is now deceased. I call the ICU.*)

Me: What happened with that patient?

ICU: Oh, he wasn't doing well. We had a family meeting and decided to withdraw care.

Me: But when did you decide that?

ICU: Oh, we turned everything off about ten minutes after you left.

Me: What? You were having a family meeting about withdrawing care as I was torturing that poor man? Why did you even call me in the first place then? You realize the last memory that man now has is me suctioning out his throat, right?

ICU: Oh yeah, sorry about that.

Intern finds me in the OR

Intern: I just got a consult from Medicine.

Me: OK, what for?

Intern: Well, the Medicine intern called it on behalf of the Cardiology team. He wasn't quite sure why he was calling.

Me: OK...

Intern: Cardiology was doing a transesophageal echo on a patient and couldn't see the heart. They wanted us to rule out air in the mediastinum.

Me: Um... what?

Intern: I said that I'd run it by you.

Me: Well, I don't understand. Why would they think the patient has air in the mediastinum? Did they perforate the esophagus and not notice? I don't know much about the human body, but I'd think if there were enough air in the chest to cause the esophagus to separate from the heart, the patient would be either very sick/dead or at the very least it'd show up on a chest X-ray. How's the patient doing?

Intern: He's apparently doing fine. And they didn't get a chest X-ray. They got a CT of the chest.

Me: And what did that show?

Intern: There's no air in the mediastinum.

Me: How about that! So why did they call us?

Intern: I'm not sure. Do you want me to call them back or go see the patient?

Me: No, no. Do nothing. Hopefully they'll realize how silly that consult was and never call us again.

TRYING TO ARRANGE FOR A PATIENT TO GO THE DENTAL CLINIC

Nurse: Doctor, patient transport says they can't take the patient to dental clinic.

Me: Why not? Are they too busy right now?

Nurse: No, they say they're not allowed to take patients to dental clinic.

Me: That seems ridiculous. They take patients to other clinics, though, right?

Nurse: Yes. They take patients to the ophthalmology clinic all the time.

(*Call patient transport and ask them why they can't transport my patient.*)

Patient transporter: Um . . . I don't know, you have to speak to my supervisor.

Supervisor: We don't transport patients to dental clinic.

Me: So what do you guys do if you don't transport patients?

Supervisor: We do transport patients. Just to certain areas. And not to dental clinic. Nursing aides do that.

Me: But why can't you do it?

Supervisor: That's the policy. It's been in place for two years. And we always get into this argument.

Me: Because it doesn't make any sense. You take patients to ophthalmology clinic all the time. That clinic is in another building altogether. You're telling me you're not allowed to take patients to the dental clinic, which is only on the bottom floor of the hospital much less in another building?

Supervisor: That's our policy. And we'd need a meeting between the head of nursing and the head of our department to change it.

Me: OK. Can you fax me a copy of that policy? I want to see where it's written that nursing aides and not patient transport are responsible for transporting patients to dental clinic.

Supervisor, *taken aback*: Wait, you want to see the policy?

Me: Yeah, I do. I want to see it in writing. 'Cause, otherwise, it sounds like you're making it up.

Supervisor: Well . . . it's not actually written down. But I'm sure it's a nursing policy.

Nurse, *has been listening to this conversation*: That's crazy. We don't have anything like that.

Me: Right.

Call from Medicine team— patient complaining of clogged feeling in his ear

Me: Did you guys look in the ear?

Medicine: No. We didn't have an otoscope.

Me: Well, find an otoscope and look in his ear first. They are available in this hospital. Find an enterprising third-year medical student.

(*Called back five minutes later.*)

Medicine: We couldn't find an otoscope.

Me: Doesn't seem like you looked too hard. But don't worry, I'm going to see this consult just to save myself some time later. But the next time we need a stethoscope, we're going to page you.

(*Go to see the patient and begin to look for the patient's chart at the nurses' station. Overhear the Hepatology team discussing a consult.*)

Hepatology attending: I don't understand. Why would the Medicine team consult us without doing liver enzymes?

Resident: I don't know.

Hepatology attending: I mean, we're hepatologists, right? How do you consult Hepatology without doing liver enzymes?

Me: The same way you consult ENT without looking in the ears, which is what I was just called for.

Hepatology attending: We didn't consult you, did we?

Me: Nah, you're safe.

(Glad to know it doesn't happen to us alone.)

Rounding on the floors. Been having a run of bad luck recently. Look down and see a bright shiny penny, heads up.

Me, *to two nurses*: Oh man, a penny! I've been having so much bad luck recently.

Nurse 1: Really?

Me: You have no idea. But maybe this penny is a good sign. A sign of things changing perhaps.

(*I pick up the penny.*)

Nurse 2: Doc, that penny actually fell off from a stretcher for a patient that has terrible C. diff infection.

Me, *dropping penny immediately*: What? Are you serious?

Nurse 2: Yeah, it's bad.

Me: You're not just messing with me, right?

Nurse 2: Nope.

(*I vigorously wash my hands. Streak of bad luck continues!*)

Page from Trauma

Trauma intern: Hey, we got this guy up here. He has a temporal bone fracture. Neurosurgery wanted to get your opinion on it.

Me: OK, is his face moving normally?

Trauma intern: Well, he's got a third cranial nerve palsy that we're treating with steroids.

Me: OK, but what about his face? Is his face moving normally?

Trauma intern: He's got a third cranial nerve palsy.

Me: You said that already, I appreciate that. What about his face?

Trauma intern: Um, it's fine.

Me: Is there anything leaking out of his ear?

Trauma intern: No.

Me: OK, if his face is moving normally and there's no CSF leaking from his ear, then there's not much I'm going to do. But I'll come by and see him.

(*Go see the patient. Eyes [third cranial nerve] moving normally. Facial paralysis more than evident.*)

Me: What the fuck!

(*I go find Trauma intern.*)

Discontinue Leeches!!
And Other Stories from an ENT's Training

Me: What were you talking about on the phone? That guy's eyes are moving fine. He has a facial nerve palsy!

Trauma intern: Yeah, I know.

Me: Wait, what do you think the third cranial nerve is?

Trauma intern: Um . . . the facial nerve?

Me: That's the seventh. Oculomotor is the third. What did you think I was asking when I asked if his face was moving normally?

Trauma intern: Oh, I thought you were asking if there were any lacerations on his face.

Me: Um . . . we're done here.

Called by Attending

Attending: Hey, you know that nosebleed lady you're supposed to take the nasal packing out of today? The family just called me and said they want to be there when you pull the packing out.

Me: Um . . . why? I'm taking out nasal packing. I'm not performing a magic trick.

Attending: I don't know. They wanted me to order a CT of the head too, but I told them if they wanted that, they could find a new ENT.

Me: OK, I'll see what I can do.

(*Go see the patient.*)

Me: I know I told you yesterday that today we were going to take out the packing, but your family called and said they want to be here.

Patient: Why do they need to be here?

Me: They don't really, but they insisted.

Patient: But you could take it out right now, though, right?

Me: Sure, but I don't want to get yelled at by your family.

Patient: What are you worried about them for? What are they going to do, spank you? They're ridiculous. I'll deal with them. Take the packing out.

Me: Oh man, I like you even more.

Consult from ICU

ICU resident: We have a guy up here that we can't get off the ventilator. He needs a tracheostomy.

Me: OK, is he stable to have the procedure?

ICU resident: Yup.

Me: Not on any pressors? Hemoglobin is OK? Platelets are OK? Not requiring a lot of PEEP or high percentage of oxygen?

ICU resident: He's completely stable to have the procedure.

Me: OK, did you talk to the family about a tracheostomy? Do they want it?

ICU resident: Um . . . yeah . . .

Me: You don't sound too confident. Are you sure you talked to the family?

ICU resident: Yeah. They're actually coming here today with a translator. They only speak Korean. Actually, if you're available, you can come get consent while the translator is here.

Me: Fine, I'll be there.

(*Go by the ICU at the allotted time and walk in on the ICU resident getting berated by the patient's family.*)

Family, *screaming in Korean via the translator*: He needs surgery? What do you mean he's going to have a hole in his neck? What are you talking about! Nobody told us about this!

Me, *to no one in particular*: Typical.

(*Walk out of the room and am followed by the ICU resident a few minutes later.*)

Me: So did you talk to the family?

ICU resident: They don't want a tracheostomy right now.

Me: And that's why you always talk to the family first.

Page from General Surgery

Gen Surg, *slightly embarrassed tone*: I'm really, really sorry, but we have a consult for you. It's for NG tube removal.

Me: Excuse me? For what now?

Gen Surg, *more embarrassed*: We can't get the NG tube out of this guy's nose.

Me: I don't understand. You can't just pull it out? Wait, you guys didn't suture it into place and forget to remove the stitch, did you?

Gen Surg: No, there's nothing holding it in. We just can't get it out. And our attending won't let us try again until you come evaluate the patient. I'm really sorry.

Me: Um . . . OK.

(*Go see the patient and happen to walk in the room the same time as the General Surgery attending finishing up with the patient.*)

Attending, *to patient*: The ENT specialist is here. He deals with this kind of thing all the time. I'll leave him to it.

Me, *thinking to myself*: Yeah, this is a really a first for me.

(*I introduce myself to the patient, grasp the NG tube, twist and pull, and it comes out. Patient effusively thanks me as I walk out of room.*)

Attending, *somewhat amazed*: It's out already? What did you do?

Me: Twist and pull. I'm outta here.

Received this picture from a General Surgery resident

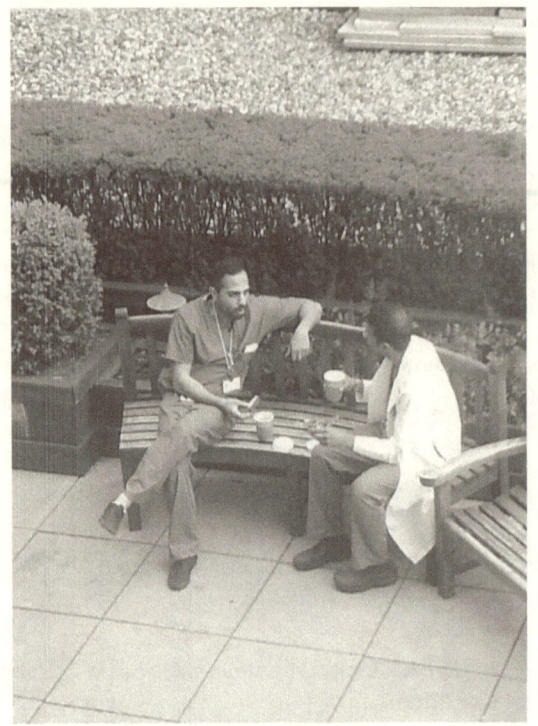

Gen Surg: Love it that you guys have date nights!

Me: Um, we're discussing patient care over coffee and biscotti. You Gen Surg people are welcome to join.

Gen Surg: Such a civilized bunch!

Me: Indeed.

Seeing patients with my attending

Attending, *looking at prescription with referral on it*: You see? I know this is going to be trouble.

(Script is from a general medical practice in the community.)

Me: I mean, has that practice sent you silly consults before?

Attending: I don't know, but I only like to get referrals from other ENTs. At least they have some idea of what's going on. Usually, when I get a referral from a general doctor, it's for some cockamamie diagnosis. You see, all they wrote on the script is "ENT referral."

Me: But look, they wrote that helpful ICD 9 code at the bottom. 307.54. We can look that up.

Attending: I suppose.

(*Attending grabs a book of ICD 9 codes from his desk. 307.54 = psychogenic vomiting.*)

Attending, *giving me a look*: I told you. It's not a promising start.

Me: All right, you got me.

Eating an egg salad sandwich in cafeteria. Sitting at the other end of the table is what appears to be a set of octogenarian Medicine attendings.

Attending 1: These residents these days! They rely too much on tests to tell them what to do! I mean, a patient has purulent secretions and decreased breath sounds on one side, he or she has pneumonia! What do they need a chest X-ray for? Just treat them!

Attending 2: I know what you mean. Residents these days can't do a proper physical exam.

Attending 3: Exactly! The other day, one of the residents said the patient had an earache. And then he didn't know how to use an otoscope.

(*All pause in reflection. Then they all look down the table at me.*)

Me, *looking up at them*: I'm an ENT resident. I know how to use an otoscope better than all of you.

(*Finish up my sandwich and leave.*)

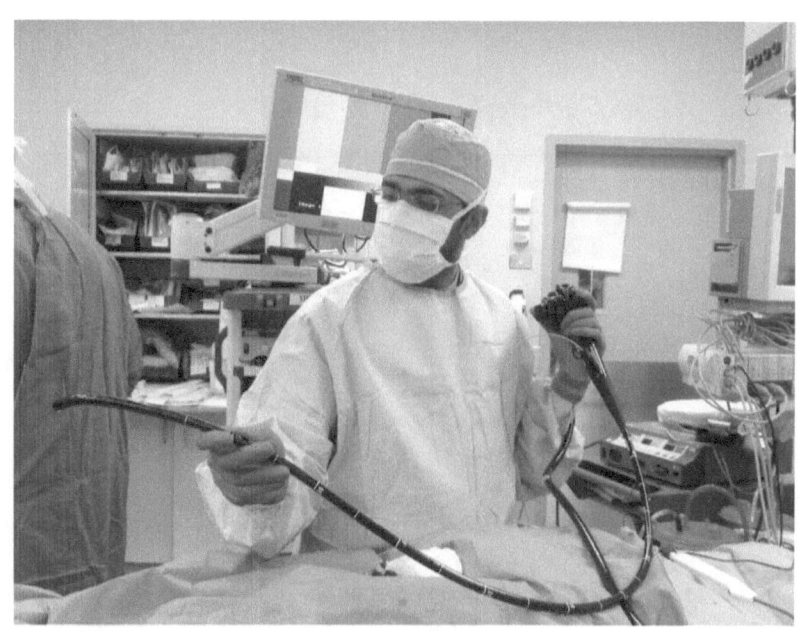

Chief Year

Junior resident gets a page. I hear only his end of conversation.

Junior: Hello? What's going on? No. No smoking! All right, bye.

Me: What was that about?

Junior: Some resident just called asking if it was all right if our patient who has cancer on his vocal cords could go outside and smoke.

Me: Wait, what?

Junior: Yeah, I know! That takes the call of the day for me.

Me: I don't understand. How does that even make any sense? You should call them back and ask them if they're really a doctor.

Junior: Oh man, I really should have yelled at them. Or given the phone to you.

Me: I would have destroyed them.

Junior: I really missed my chance.

Me: Yeah, you really did.

Going through cases for the next day with new third-year medical student

Me: Oh, I have a robot/neck tomorrow.

Student: You're doing robotic surgery on the neck? That's cool!

Me: Nah, all that means is that we're using the robot to remove a tumor from someone's mouth and then doing a neck dissection.

Student, *somewhat perplexed*: Robot/neck? That's an odd way of referring to it though.

Me: Well, as surgeons, we tend to communicate things in the most abbreviated format possible. "Transoral robotic surgery" becomes "robot," "thyroidectomy" becomes "thyroid," "tympanoplasty with possible mastoidectomy" becomes "T-mastoid," and such and such. For example, when I say to another resident, "Hey, you're doing a tranny tomorrow," it means that they are doing an endoscopic transsphenoidal resection of a pituitary mass with neurosurgery, not that they are operating on a transsexual patient.

Student: Um . . .

Me: Don't worry, you'll catch on. Then you'll move to another service and have to learn a whole new language. Welcome to Surgery.

SETTING UP FOR ENDOSCOPIC SINUS SURGERY CASE

Me: All right, do we have all the equipment? Can we say the room is ready and bring the patient back?

Circulator: Almost, we're just waiting on the endoscopes.

(*Equipment tech arrives with tray labeled "sinus endoscopy."*)

Me: All right, let's open it up and make sure they have the thirty-degree scope. We'll need it for this case.

(*They open the tray to reveal a Bookwalter retractor.*)

Me, *staring a good ten seconds*: So that's a Bookwalter retractor. That's for open abdomen surgery and not for sinus surgery.

Equipment tech: Oh, you can't use that?

Me: Well, unless you want me doing some sort of exploratory laparotomy on this guy, then, no. I don't particularly want to look in his belly. I only want to look in his nose.

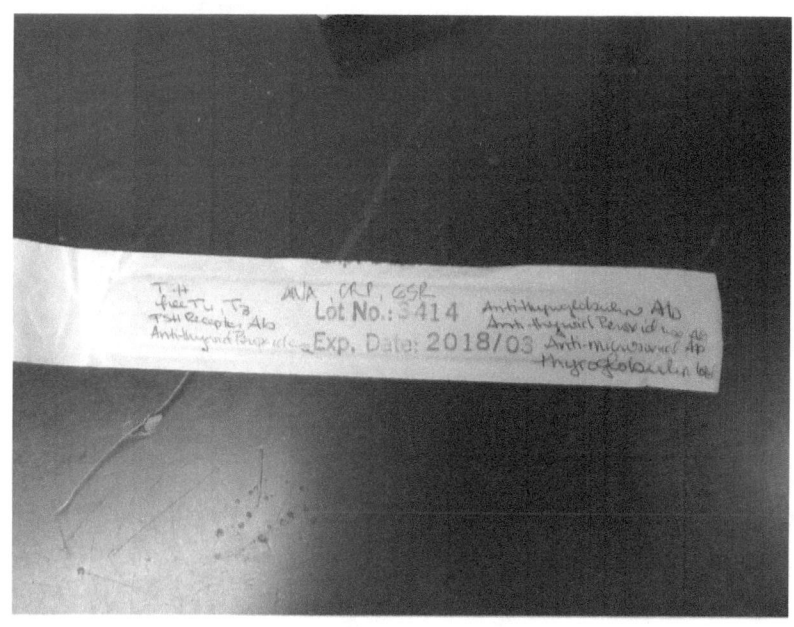

DISCUSSING A PATIENT WE'RE ABOUT TO TAKE TO OR WITH ATTENDING

Attending: Yeah, we should just get some repeat labs before taking the patient to the OR.

(*Attending grabs a tongue blade from white coat and starts writing furiously.*)

Me: Um, do you want maybe a piece of paper?

Attending: Nah, this is fine.

(*Hands me the pictured tongue blade.*)

Attending: Make sure all these are drawn. Some are send out labs, so just call the lab to make sure you know the correct colored tubes for each specimen. And do it as quickly as possible. I want to start the case in fifteen minutes.

Me: Uh . . .

Attending: And you can keep the tongue blade.

Me: Thanks?

SEEING A PATIENT WITH LOUD STRIDOR AND RETRACTIONS

Me: We have to look at your airway through your nose.

Patient: (*Gasp*) What? (*Gasp*) OK!

(*Scope the patient and find a giant tumor obstructing her larynx.*)

Me: OK. You have a large mass blocking off your airway. We need to take you to the OR and do a tracheostomy, essentially put a breathing tube into your neck. But we need to do it awake because if we put you to sleep, you'll completely close off your airway and you'll stop breathing.

Patient: (*Gasp*) Am (*gasp*) I (*gasp*) going (*gasp*) to (*gasp*) be (*gasp*) all right? (*Gasp*)

(*Longer than normal pause on my part as I consider all the airway disasters possible. Also use the time to make sure I have a scalpel ready in my pocket.*)

Me: You're going to be fine.

Patient: (*Gasp*) Why (*gasp*) did (*gasp*) you (*gasp*) take (*gasp*) so (*gasp*) long (*gasp*) to (*gasp*) answer? (*Gasp*)

(*Junior resident nearly cracks up laughing.*)

Me: No, I didn't. You'll be fine. No more talking now. We're going to get you upstairs as soon as possible.

Junior resident: You did take a long time to answer her.

(*The junior resident and I leave to go up to the OR to prepare the case. The junior resident turns to me.*)

Me: Well, shit, the way she's breathing, she could crap out real soon. Then we're doing a cric, and it's a fucking disaster. That possibility crossed my mind. Let's just get her up there so I can keep my promise.

Talking to same day surgery nurses

Nurse 1: So, doc, how much longer do you have?

Me: Nine months. Actually, this is my last day here at this hospital for three months.

Nurse 2: Where are you going?

Me: To the VA through December. But I'll be back for my last hurrah starting in January.

Nurse 3: So what chief is coming now?

Me: Alejandro's coming back.

(*Collective "Awwwww" from nurses.*)

Nurse 2: Ale-Alejandro! We love Alejandro!

Me: So I'm curious. Do you guys have the same reaction when Alejandro tells you I'm coming back?

Nurse 1: Sure, doc, we love you too.

Me: Hmmmmm . . . if you say so.

Having a drink with some general surgeons

Gen Surg resident 1: So your Facebook profile recently has just been a bunch of pictures of food. When are you going to get back to the stories?

Me: Well, I'm a chief now, so I'm not really on the front lines or in the trenches, what have you, so I don't get the really crazy stories anymore. It's mostly my junior residents.

Gen Surg resident 2: Plus, you keep most of those stories under wraps for months.

Gen Surg resident 1: I don't care about what food you're eating. I enjoy your stories.

Me: All right, all right, I have a few stories waiting in the wings.

Gen Surg resident 1: Good.

Attending tells me we need another hand for surgery, so I decide to ask a favor from General Surgery via text.

Me: Do you have any med students right now who are superexcited about ENT?

Gen Surg resident: Unclear if a superexcited med student exists anymore.

Me: How about a med student with eyes and arms who can retract and watch a face while I do a parotidectomy tomorrow?

Gen Surg resident: Sure. I'll text the intern to let them know.

Me: Ooh, really? Let 'em know lunch may be included.

Gen Surg resident: No need to spoil them!

Me: Well, it's a pretty shitty job.

Gen Surg resident: They are med students. They know they are there to retract.

Me: All right. Maybe I'll be really, really mean to them tomorrow. See if I can make them cry.

Gen Surg resident: I'm sure you can be mean!

SEEING A WORLD WAR II VETERAN

Me: Hello, sir, what brings you in today?

Patient: I got Eustachian tube dysfunction!

Me: OK. Why do you say that?

Patient: Well, that's what they told me in Anzio when we were going up the boot! They never used to equalize the pressure in the planes when were going up and down like they do nowadays. We all had problems with our ears! But I pop my ears these days, and they're just fine!

Me: Did you ever rupture your eardrums or have any surgeries on your ears?

Patient: All I know is that one day I came down, and I was laid up in bed in Italy for a month! What do you think they did to me?

Me: I'm sorry, sir, I don't particularly know what they did or didn't do to your ears in a hospital in Italy seventy years ago.

Patient, *laughing*: I suppose not. Isn't it in your idiot box over there? (*Gestures to my computer.*)

Me: Nah, unfortunately the records don't go back that far.

Patient: I don't know why. They had computers back then too. Well, that's my story. I'm hearing just fine today.

(*Examine patient. Ears and eardrums are normal.*)

Me: Well, your ears look normal today. But I believe you when you tell me this is a problem. I could put tubes in your eardrums so you don't have to keep popping your ears.

Discontinue Leeches!!
And Other Stories from an ENT's Training

Patient: No, I don't want any surgery! I'm ninety years old! I'm fine! In fact, I don't know why I came today. I just got a letter in the mail telling me to be here, so here I am!

Me: Fair enough, you're free to go. Thank you for your service.

(WW II vets are the BEST!)

Call from Fast Track

Nurse: We have this patient here, and I'm pretty sure he has a tumor in his right ear. I mean, I'm looking in there, and it looks bizarre. I've never seen anything like it. It has to be cancer.

Me: OK. We have clinic right now, so send him up.

(*Patient comes up to clinic, sits in the chair, and looks really uncomfortable.*)

Me: Sir, I hear you've been having some issues with your right ear. How long has that been going on for?

Patient: Since last night.

Me: Hm. And everything was fine before then?

Patient: Yeah. I can't hear anything out of it now, and it feels funny.

Me: Let's have a look.

(*Look in right ear and see a cockroach, which is fortunately dead.*)

Me: You have a cockroach in your ear.

Patient: Really? Well, my sister has been having a problem with them.

(*I fish it out and show the patient.*)

Patient: Oh man, I gotta move!

Me: Advisable.

Discontinue Leeches!!
And Other Stories from an ENT's Training

(*Call back Fast Track.*)

Me: So it was actually a cockroach.

Nurse: No way! That was definitely a tumor.

Me: Well, it had a thorax and legs, so I'm gonna go with cockroach.

SEEING A PATIENT COMPLAINING OF LIQUID COMING OUT OF HIS NOSE WHEN SWALLOWING

Patient: Yeah, it's really annoying, and it happens with water.

Me: Hm. Have you ever had surgery on your tonsils? Or surgery for sleep apnea? Like soft palate surgery?

Patient: Well, I had my tonsils removed when I was a kid, but nothing else.

(Look through his chart and see that repeated swallowing tests have been normal.)

Me: It looks like all the studies have been normal.

Patient: Yeah, it never happens when I do the test. Typical.

Me: Can you show me what happens?

Patient: Sure.

(Give the patient a cup of water. He takes a gulp of water, turns his head nearly upside down, coughs, and then tries to swallow. Water comes out of his nose.]

Me: Um, what are you doing?

Patient: This is when it happens, when I bend over like this!

Me: Uh, do you usually try to swallow like that?

Patient: Nah, when I'm sitting upright, there's no problem. It's only when I try to swallow with my head turned over that it happens.

Me: OK. Don't do that.

Patient: But what's causing it?

Me: You are. I could make water come out of my nose if I did that.

Patient: Really? I thought something was wrong.

Me: I wouldn't worry about it.

DOING A LARGE COMPOSITE RESECTION FOR CANCER. GET TO THE POINT IN THE OPERATION WHERE ENTIRE SPECIMEN INCLUDING PART OF THE JAW, FLOOR OF MOUTH, AND TONGUE ARE ABOUT TO COME OUT IN ONE PIECE.

Me, *shaking my head*: Hmmmm . . .

Attending: What is it? You find something amusing?

Me: Not really. But I mean, do you ever just step back and think what in God's name are we doing? It's crazy the stuff we do here!

Attending: Yeah, you're right. Without a medical license, in some states, we'd get the chair for this. All right, let's get this tumor out.

Patient on OR table, about to be induced for anesthesia

Russian anesthesiologist: Sir, we are going to give you some oxygen.

Patient: Where's the doctor?

Anesthesiologist: You mean the surgeon? He's on his way right now. Let me give you this oxygen.

Patient: You're not putting that mask on me! Knock me out! I want the doctor!

Anesthesiologist: Are you here to get an operation? Or are you here to give me a hard time?

Patient: You can knock me out first! But don't put that mask on me until you do! I want a doctor!

Anesthesiologist: I am a doctor! This is America! We don't knock people out! We give them general anesthesia! Give me propofol!

Discharging a patient after operating on him for epistaxis

Patient: I can't thank you enough for what you did. By the way, this is my friend.

(*Patient gestures to the other man in the room.*)

Me: Nice to meet you. So you're going to have to be really careful at home. We don't want you blowing your nose.

Patient: At all?

Me: At all. It can put stress on all the little blood vessels in your nose and cause you to bleed again.

Friend: So the doc is saying the only blowing you'll be doing is when you're blowing me!

Patient: Haha! Exactly!

Me: Um . . . moving on, no heavy lifting, and try not to bend over at all, if you can help it.

Friend: So, doc, can I still bend him over the toilet?

(*Awkward pause.*)

Patient: Ha! Exactly!

Me: Nah, I'd recommend against that. On that happy note, we'll see you in a couple of weeks.

Patient: Did you just say "on that happy note"?

Me: I did.

Patient: Oh man, I like you, doc!

Late night e-mail from attending

"I have a meeting tomorrow afternoon for about an hour so please see the pt's and send them out. I'll get there as soon as I can. If a patient insists on my seeing them, I'll do so when I get there."

(Attending's clinic is particularly long with a lot of patients to see, and we are usually there from 1:00 PM to 6:00–7:30 PM seeing patients with him.)

Me, *to team, on the morning of clinic*: Guys, we have an opportunity here. We're going to absolutely destroy clinic today. We will see as many patients as is humanly possible before he gets to clinic and send them out, and we're going to finish clinic early or at least on time today.

(*Start clinic at one. By two, we've seen seventeen patients and sent them out. Attending shows up, and it takes three hours to see the last thirteen patients.*)

Attending, *at five fifteen, looking around*: Wow. Are we done with clinic already?

Me: Absolutely.

Attending: Huh. I should not show up to my clinic more often!

Finishing up a case in the OR

Nurse: What was your diagnosis for the patient?

Me: Chronic sinusitis.

Nurse: And what was the procedure done?

Me: Bilateral maxillary antrostomy, total ethmoidectomy, and frontal sinusotomy.

Nurse, *writing them down*: OK, OK, and frontal sodomy?

Me: Not frontal sodomy. Frontal sinusotomy, with a *t*. We don't sodomize people here.

Nurse: Oh OK, OK.

GRAND ROUNDS. ATTENDING WALKS IN AND REALIZES THERE'S NO SIGN-IN SHEET.

Attending 1: Oh, uh, hey, Amit, I see there's no sign-in sheet.

Me: Yes.

Attending 1: Um, which resident is supposed to be in charge of that?

Me: Well, usually, it's your secretary who prints those things out, but if you want to make it a resident job, we can do that.

Attending 1, *clearly disappointed in my response*: Yeah, you're chief resident, you should be on top of these things.

Me: OK.

(*Later, computer the presenter is using decides to auto-update and begin a countdown to automatic restart.*)

Attending 2: Hey, Amit, why is the computer updating like that? Can you take care of that?

Me: I don't know, but I'll get a laptop.

Attending 2: Why does it have to auto-update in the middle of the presentation?

Me: I don't know. It's on the hospital network, so who knows what they have it doing?

(*Attending 2 shakes head, disappointed in my response.*)

(*Even later, presenter is using the department-issued laser pointer.*)

Discontinue Leeches!!
And Other Stories from an ENT's Training

Attending 3: Do you have a laser pointer he can use?

Me: No. But he's using the department one.

Attending 3: Why isn't it working?

Me: It is working. It just doesn't work very well.

Attending 3, *disappointed in my response*: You should do something about that.

Me: OK.

Finishing up a case in the OR

Nurse: Hey, doc, what's the name of the specimen?

Me: Right nasal alar lesion.

Nurse: Right anal lesion?

Me: Nope. Alar, a-l-a-r. The ENT service doesn't do anal. That'll be General Surgery. Or GI.

Nurse: Oh! Sorry, doc.

Me: No worries.

Entering orders on a patient with another resident at the VA

Resident: I'm gonna put him on ceftriaxone for the infection. Let's put him on Metamucil as well.

(*Resident signs orders. Warning pops up.*)

Warning: Patient has reported previous reaction to dextrose. Please provide justification in box below. (Dextrose is listed as ingredient in Metamucil and ceftriaxone.)

(*Resident writes in justification box "yourmom" and then signs order.*)

Me: Wait, did you just write "your mom" as a justification to Pharmacy?

Resident, *laughs*: Oh shoot, did I? That's actually my signature code. I do that a lot. Well, it's ridiculous anyway. The guy's been on D5 (5% dextrose) since he's been here!

Me: I'm sure the Pharmacy appreciates that.

SEEING PATIENTS IN CLINIC

Me, *to nurse*: You can send Mr. Smith back.

Nurse, *shaking her head*: Oh man, Mr. Smith . . .

Me: Is there something I should be worried about?

Nurse: Nah, he's just crazy.

Me: Perfect.

(*Look through old records, patient's been seen for ear discharge and oily skin by nearly every service in the hospital, including Psychiatry. Our last note documents that his ears are clear and that he has oily skin.*)

Me: What brings you in here today?

Patient: Doc, I got all this oil coming out of my ears! And my skin! It feels like sandpaper sometimes, and it's oily sometimes. Especially on my belly!

(*Look the patient over and look in his ears, which are normal. Skin is slightly oily.*)

Me: OK, well, your ears look clear. The drums are normal, and there's no fluid. Your skin is a bit oily. But I don't think anything dangerous is going on.

Patient: Then what's all the stuff coming out of my ears?

Me: It could just be wax. Your body produces it, and it can naturally come out of your ears. It's a normal process. As for the oily skin over your entire body, I can send you to Dermatology. I don't think you need to come back here.

Patient: I don't believe you. Your ears don't clean themselves.

Discontinue Leeches!!
And Other Stories from an ENT's Training

Me: They do though. It's normal.

Patient: I can't understand you.

Me: I'm sorry, sometimes I speak a little softly. (*In a louder voice*) Your ears clean themselves naturally.

Patient: I can hear you! I just can't understand you with that accent! Where are you from?

Me: Um, what? I'm from western New York. And I don't think I have an accent.

Patient: No, no, no. Not where you came to, where you were born! Where were you born?

Me: Buffalo, New York.

Patient: God. Why do I keep coming here? I've been here seven times, and you always tell me the same thing. None of you people do anything! You could do your job over the telephone. The telephone!

Me: You don't have to come back here, that's what I'm telling you. There's nothing wrong with your ears.

Patient: So now what? Do I have to come back here?

Me: No. You may leave.

(*Patient walks out of clinic muttering under his breath about immigrants.*)

Waiting for a case to go to the OR. Things seem to be taking a long time.

Me, *to OR front desk*: What's going on with my room?

Front desk: We're waiting for turnover.

Me: But the last case finished two hours ago. I mean, the patient is already down here. What's taking so long?

Front desk: But the last patient had an infection, so they have to really clean the room well.

Me: But it never takes this long. And a lot of our patients have infections. What was it? MRSA? VRE? MDR Klebsiella?

Front desk, *leaning over and whispering*: Worse. Bed bugs.

(*Long pause.*)

Me: What?

Front desk, *still whispering*: The last patient had bed bugs. They're steam cleaning the room right now.

Me, *leaning in and whispering*: So . . . you're telling me that for patients that have straight-up tuberculosis, it takes about half an hour to turn over the room, while patients with bed bugs triggers some sort of massive alarm where it takes two hours to turn over? Also, why are we whispering?

Front desk: I don't want bed bugs! Do you want bed bugs?

Me: Not particularly. But I don't want tuberculosis either. Whatever, call me when the room is ready, I guess.

Seeing patients in clinic. Patient comes in after radiation therapy to the neck for cancer.

Patient: I can't turn my head to the left.

Me: I'm really sorry about that. It's because of the radiation. It's very good at killing cancer, but unfortunately, it can sometimes cause a lot of scarring that interferes with the muscles. I can refer you to Physical Therapy to see if stretching the area helps break up the scar tissue.

Patient: OK. But I can't turn my head to the left.

Me: Um . . . again, I'm sorry about that. It's because of the radiation, like I explained.

Patient: So it's the radiation?

Me: Yes.

Patient: But I can't turn my head to the left.

(*This goes on for about ten minutes.*)

Me: OK. Take this sheet up to the front, and they'll take care of checking you out.

Patient: But I have something else that maybe you could help me with.

Me: OK . . .

(*Patient pulls out a folder from his bag, rummages around in it, and pulls out a credit card statement.*)

Patient: Why is there this charge here?

(Charge is from a Holiday Inn in Boca Raton.)

Me, *stare at him blankly for about ten seconds*: I don't know. You should take this up with your credit card company.

Patient: But why is the charge there?

Me: So this is an ear, nose, and throat clinic. I cannot help you with your credit card problems.

Patient: Well, who in this hospital can pay for this?

Me: Probably no one. You have to call the credit card company.

Patient: But I did. And they took away my credit card.

Me: OK, you need to go now. You need to call your credit card company. I literally cannot help you with this.

BACK IN CLINIC. SEEING A SEVENTY-SIX-YEAR-OLD MAN FOR HEARING LOSS.

Me: What brings you in here today?

Patient: I can't hear well out of my right ear.

Me: How long has it been going for?

Patient: Son, let me give you some history. I had a big surgery on my ear right ear when I was five years old. They removed all the bone from behind the ear 'cause it kept draining out.

Me: So you've had hearing loss for seventy-one years?

Patient: Well, yeah. Sort of. I think so. Also, a grenade went off by my head in 1961, and I've had worsening hearing loss ever since then.

Me: OK. Anything else happen since then? Did you have a lot of noise exposure, say, in your job?

Patient: I worked around steam engines and whistles every day for forty years. Does that count?

Me: I'd say yes. So what can I help you with today?

Patient: I want the army to compensate me for my hearing loss now because of the grenade from 1961. I need a doctor to say that all my hearing loss is from the grenade.

Me: Um . . . I can't do that.

Patient: Well, my private ENT gave me a hearing test and said that all my hearing loss is because of the grenade.

Me: OK. I'm not gonna lie to you. I think your hearing loss is probably from all three of those things combined at the very least. Also, it's a bit silly for me to comment on a grenade explosion from over fifty years ago, particularly if you had ear disease and surgery before that, and you were exposed to loud whistles for forty years afterward.

Patient: Well, why did my other doctor tell me it was all from the grenade?

Me: I don't know why he said that.

Patient: All right, sonny, you write what you need to write. Thank you for being honest. I'm going to have a word or two with this other guy.

Operating with Attending, also the Chair of the Department, taking out a Parotid Gland Tumor

Me: Do you mind if I put on my music?

Attending: No, go ahead.

Me: It's a pretty varied mix of stuff.

Attending: OK.

(*While dissecting along the facial nerve, music switches from "Rhapsody in Blue" to the Icona Pop song "I Love It." Several key moves are made while the lyrics "I love it! I don't care! I love it!" are being sung. Song ends.*)

Attending: So you did a good job, but if it were me, I wouldn't have picked that song to dissect out the facial nerve.

Me: Really?

Attending: I can't dissect anything when there's a back beat! I feel like I should be in a club somewhere. Maybe something a bit more laid-back next time? Your music is so schizophrenic! I mean, it's nice you have such varied tastes, but I can't tell what's coming next!

Me: I did warn you.

Attending: You did.

Talking to General Surgery resident regarding Trauma call early in her rotation earlier this year

Me: How was call?

Resident: Call was uneventful.

Me: Good way to ease into things I guess. Time to prepare yourself for the nonsense.

Resident: That's how I took it. Plenty of time left on the rotation for an ED thoracotomy.

Me: True story. Hopefully not the norm for you. By the way, when I get around to writing a living will, it's going to say: "In the event of me needing an ED thoracotomy, just let me fucking die."

Resident: But how will budding Trauma surgeons learn? In all seriousness.

Me: All right, I'll put in a corollary for if there are residents present. So long as afterward, if it looks like I'm circling the drain, someone can "accidentally" terminally extubate me.

(Gotta do what you gotta do to become a good surgeon.)

About to start a free flap case. On positioning the patient, we discover the patient also has a large abscess on his upper back.

Anesthesia attending: You need to call your attending about this. This is something we might have to cancel the case for.

Me: OK . . .

(*Call attending into room. He stares at the abscess.*)

Attending: We need to call General Surgery. Amit, call General Surgery.

Me: Are you kidding? It's an abscess. On his back. It's practically bursting through the skin.

Attending: What do you want to do?

Me: I'm not going to call General Surgery for this! We should just drain it. It'll be quicker, and if General Surgery has taught me anything, it's how to drain an abscess. They put up with a lot of nonsense from us. I know for a fact that they will laugh us out of the room if we call them for this.

Attending: Fine.

Finish up my last case of my residency, a modified radical neck dissection for cancer. Drop the patient off in the ICU with the second-year General Surgery resident, who's running the unit.

Me: OK, so he had a neck dissection, We took the jugular but left the SCM and accessory spinal. He has moderate COPD but no other issues. Shouldn't give you any issues overnight.

Resident: OK, great, we'll keep an eye on him.

(*Finish a few things up and then start heading home. Get a call from the resident.*)

Resident: I just coded your patient.

Me: What? What happened?

Resident: Don't know. We're trying to figure that out.

Me: OK, I'll be there in a bit.

(*Call my attending, and we arrive around the same time.*)

Resident: He just started desaturating all of a sudden and then coded. We reintubated him, did CPR, got him back. Labs are pending.

Me: Well, nice job!

Resident: That was my first solo code.

Me: You did an awesome job! And that was my last case here.

Resident: Really?

Me: Really.

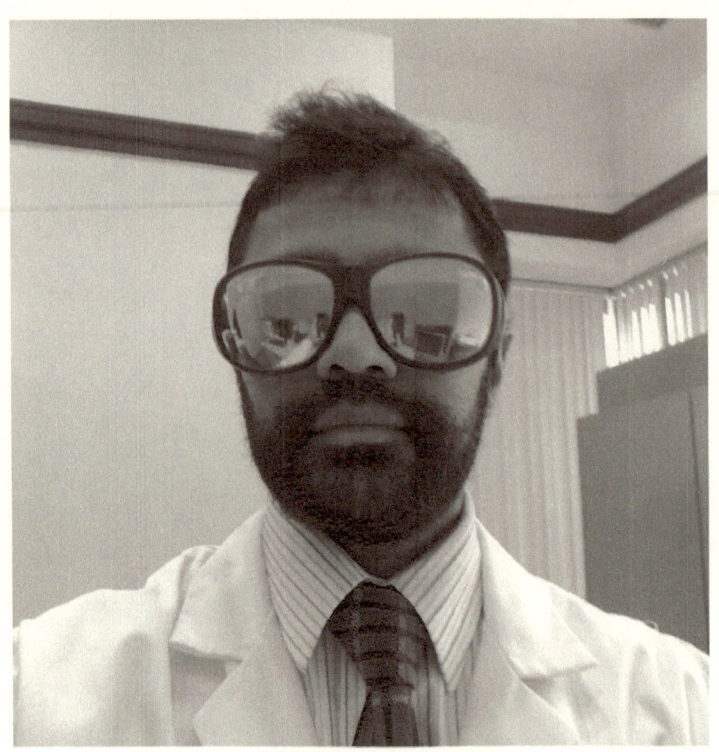

Fellowship

New Hospital Bureaucracy—trying to get access to the electronic medical record system. Call placed to IT.

Me: So I was able to generate a username and password, but when I put it into the EMR training site, it says it's incorrect.

Tech: Um . . . did you activate you account through central processing?

Me: No, let me try.

(*Go to the website he indicates, enter in my social security number and date of birth, only to have it tell me it doesn't recognize me.*)

Tech: Hm . . . it says in my system your employment was terminated.

Me: That makes no sense. I've only been here six days. How was it terminated? Also, I have an employee number, and I got an ID today.

Tech: So Security issues the ID badges. They're separate from HR, which is also separate from IT.

Me: So I can walk into the hospital but can't do anything there.

Tech: Yeah. So you need to call HR.

(*Call placed to HR.*)

HR: It says here your application is incomplete.

Me: I've submitted all the forms multiple times. HR gave me an employee number. What else do I have to do?

HR: Do you have a life number?

Me: I don't know what that is.

HR: It's a number given to you by us. You don't have to know what it is, only if you have one or not.

Me: You should be able to tell me that, I think, if you're the ones who assign these life numbers.

HR: Yeah, you don't have a life number.

Me: Right. Can you give me one?

HR: It's going to have to be done tomorrow. The computers are busy with payroll today.

Me: Are you messing with me? All the computers you have are busy with payroll? This is really going to become a patient care issue. I'm on call tomorrow and will need access, say, in case there's some sort of emergency and I might want to write orders on a patient.

HR: Oh, it'll be done tomorrow. It only takes twenty-four to forty-eight hours of processing.

Me: So how will it be done tomorrow if it you're going to do it tomorrow and then it takes another one to two days after that to process it?

HR: It'll probably be done.

Me: Probably? Perfect.

FIRST WEEKEND TAKING CALL AS A FELLOW. BEEN ROCKING A REASONABLY HEAVY BEARD IN THE HOPES THAT IT MAKES ME LOOK SOMEWHAT MORE AUTHORITATIVE. GET CALLED TO SCOPE A PATIENT FOR POSSIBLE AIRWAY SWELLING.

Me: My name is Dr. Patel, I'm an ENT doctor. They called me because you felt like your airway was closing up.

Patient, *somewhat anxious*: Yeah, that's right. I ate a tomato earlier and I broke out, and it felt like I was going to suffocate. So I took my epi pen.

Me: So you're allergic to tomatoes. Has this happened to you before?

Patient: Five times this year. But I always take my epi pen, and it goes away.

Me: Um . . . this only happens when you eat tomatoes?

Patient: Yes.

Me: Hm. You should probably stop eating tomatoes. Anyway, you're here now, so I have to look at your airway. The way I do that is with a small scope that goes through your nose so I can see your voice box.

Patient, *really anxious*: You know, you look awfully young.

Me: What?

Patient: You look so young! Are you sure you've done this before?

Me: Many, many times. I'm just surprised you think I look young. I mean, you should see me without this beard! I look like I'm twelve years old.

Patient, *suddenly mortified*: Oh, doctor, I didn't mean to offend you! I'm so sorry.

Me: Don't worry, it takes a lot to offend me.

Patient, *still mortified*: I really didn't want to offend you though. Are you still going to help me?

Me: It's my job. OK, let's make a deal. I won't be offended if you promise to stop eating tomatoes.

Patient: OK, OK. Thank you. Do you still have to put that thing in my nose?

Me: Oh yeah.

Called for possible airway swelling

ER: There's this lady down here. She took a Tylenol today, and now she has hives, and her voice might be a bit raspy.

Me: OK. How does she look? Any stridor?

ER: She looks comfortable. No stridor. We called Anesthesia to look at her.

Me, *a bit taken aback*: Why'd you call Anesthesia? You think she needs to be intubated?

ER: We figured you weren't in house, so we wanted someone to evaluate her airway.

Me: OK. So what did they say?

ER: They said they can't evaluate the airway.

Me: What does that mean?

ER: They said they can't evaluate the airway until ENT scopes her.

Me: But they're anesthesiologists. A significant portion of their jobs revolves around evaluating airways.

ER: Yeah, they said they can't.

Me: That seems silly. Anyone can assess an airway, particularly an anesthesiologist. I can understand if they evaluated her and said they needed me to scope the patient, but whatever, I'll come and see her.

(*Go to ER, find the patient lying flat in bed, playing Candy Crush. I ask her to open her mouth, and I can see her epiglottis. Voice does sound a bit raspy.*)

Me: Ma'am, has your voice changed?

Patient: Nope, this is my normal voice.

Me: All right, I'm outta here.

ER: Wait, do you want to talk to Anesthesia?

Me: Nah, I don't think I'd be very nice to them.

Seeing patients in my clinic

Me: What brings you to the clinic today?

Patient: The inside of my ear was really itching a few days ago, so I started scratching it. It started bleeding, and I got really scared, so I went to the urgent care place. They gave me antibiotics and told me to come here.

Me: What were you scratching it with?

Patient: Whatever was there. You know, a stick.

Me: Like a Q-tip?

Patient: No, no. Like one of those sticks!

Me: Um . . . from a tree?

Patient: Stick! Like the ones that come with food.

Me: Uh . . . a toothpick?

Patient: Nah, man, like the Chinese food!

Me: A chopstick! You were scratching your ear with a chopstick?

Patient: Yeah, yeah, chopstick! It worked really well until the bleeding.

Me: Well, you shouldn't put anything in your ears.

Patient: I'll never use chopsticks again.

Me: No, not just chopsticks. Don't put anything in your ears! Nothing!

Patient, *crestfallen*: Oh.

Consult for ringing in the ears

Me: It says here you have ringing in your ears.

Patient: Yeah, it's like a clicking noise. I got it real bad in both ears.

Me: Does it sound like your heartbeat?

Patient: Yeah, it does.

Me: It's definitely in time with your heartbeat? It's not a ringing or buzzing sound, is it?

Patient: No, it's like a ringing and buzzing too!

Me: So it's all three?

Patient: Yeah, sometimes it's like my heart, sometimes it's ringing, sometimes it's buzzing.

Me: Hm. Can you make the noise for me?

(*Patient starts smacking his lips.*)

Patient, *in between lip smacks*: That's what it's like.

Me: Uh . . . that doesn't sound like anything you described.

Patient: Yeah, but it's like that. Like a smacking!

Me: OK. Do you have drainage from your ears?

Patient: All the time.

Discontinue Leeches!!
And Other Stories from an ENT's Training

Me: Any feeling of vertigo, like the room spinning with nausea? Or feeling like you're going to pass out?

Patient: Man, I'm dizzy all the time! I'm always about to pass out.

Me: How about hearing loss?

Patient: I feel like I'm completely deaf. It's terrible.

Me: But you can hear me now.

Patient: I'm not deaf now.

Me: All right, let me examine you.

(Entire exam is normal.)

Me: OK, the first step is a hearing test. I'll order it for you, and when you come back, we can talk about what to do next.

Patient: What about painkillers?

Me: What about them?

Patient: Aren't you going to give me any oxy? My neck is killing me. (*Starts rolling his neck around on his shoulders.*)

Me: No. You can have a hearing test. But no painkillers.

Patient: Really? Oh whatever.

Seeing patients in my clinic

Me: It says here you're here for nosebleeds.

Patient: Yeah, but I should have cancelled this appointment. I figured out what was wrong. I was having nosebleeds on and off a couple of years ago, nothing too serious.

Me: So what happened?

Patient: I stopped drinking Coors Light.

(*Silence.*)

Patient: Well, I don't know if it was that I stopped drinking Coors Light from bottles or that I started drinking Heineken from cans.

Me: OK, Let me just take a look in your nose and make sure nothing is really going on.

(Nose is clear.)

Patient: So, doc, what do you think it was?

Me: I have no idea. The only way to figure it out is to go back to Coors Light and see if you have nosebleeds again.

Patient: I don't want to do that.

Me: Yeah, me neither. You may go.

Patient: Thanks!

Seeing a patient with my attending

Attending: The reason your voice is bad is because one of the vocal cord is paralyzed. You have a few options, and it's based completely on your symptoms. We can observe, we can inject the vocal cord, or we can do a surgery to move the vocal cord over.

Patient: What do you think I should do?

Attending: Again, it's based on your symptoms. We've done a pretty extensive workup, and there's no identifiable cause. So if you're all right with your voice, we don't have to do anything.

Patient: But I leave the decision to you.

Attending: But it's your choice.

(*Patient turns to me and winks.*)

Patient: You're Italian, right?

Me: Uh . . . no. No one's ever thought I was Italian.

Patient: Yeah, Patel, that's an Italian name. What do you think I should do?

Attending, *joking*: Yeah, he's probably from those southern parts of Sicily.

Me: Well, I have to agree with my attending. If your voice is interfering with your life, then we can do one of the two procedures. If not, we don't have to do anything.

Patient: You're not giving me any answers! What should I do?

Attending: You need to give us some guidance so we can help you.

(*Patient gets up and storms out. A little while later, one of the nurses come up to us.*)

Nurse, *confused*: You saw this patient before, right? She keeps asking for the Italian doctor. Do you know who that is?

Me: Me, I guess.

Attending: Wait, she was being serious? What did she think, his name was Patelli and they changed it at Ellis Island?

Nurse: We were so confused.

Attending: I hate crazy people.

Me: Yup.

Eating my birthday cake that the office staff got for me

Nursing assistant: This cake reminds me of you.

Me: Sweet and brown?

Nursing assistant: Tan and white. Your skin is tanned, and you're wearing a white coat.

Me: You know this isn't a tan, right? It's my skin color.

Nursing assistant: I'm from the Ukraine, so my English is not so good. I mean your skin is tan colored. Anyway, happy birthday!

Me: Awesome. Thanks!

IN THE OR

Nurse: What setting do you want the laser at? Five watts?

Me: 1.21 gigawatts.

(*Anesthesiologist cracks up but stifles it.*)

Nurse: What? How much?

Me: 1.21 gigawatts. Like "jigga" watts.

Nurse: I don't think it goes that high.

Me: No? All right, five watts then.

(*Anesthesiologist loses it completely.*)

SEEING PATIENTS IN MY CLINIC

Me: Hello, sir, what brings you here today?

Patient: I'm here for my allergies. My face swelled up, and I went to the ER. They gave me some medications, and it went away.

Me: OK, what do you think you're allergic to?

Patient: Well, I know what I'm allergic to! It's the skin of the plantain. My lover made me some plantains the other day, but he didn't cook them right, and he left the skins on, and my face swelled up.

Me: All right, that makes sense.

Patient: But I've had plantains all my life, but the cooked ones! I have no problems with those.

Me: That's pretty common. Some people are allergic just to the skins of fruit but not the fruit itself. It happens with bananas, avocados, and kiwis. It's related to latex allergy. Any sensitivity to latex?

Patient: Man, I got twenty-five kids and a bunch of baby mamas. If I were allergic to latex, my dick would have fallen off a long time ago.

(*Long pause.*)

Me: Fair enough, let's move on.

DELI ACROSS FROM HOSPITAL RUNS OUT OF SPLENDA. DECIDE TO GO TO THE HOSPITAL CAFETERIA TO GET SOME. AM CONFRONTED BY A NURSE AT THE ENTRANCE OF THE HOSPITAL ASKING ABOUT FLU SHOTS.

Nurse: Did you get a flu shot? I don't see a sticker on your ID saying you did.

Me: I did get a flu shot. The sticker is on the back of my ID.

(*Turn over ID, showing a sticker from the flu shot vial with the details of the vaccine.*)

Nurse: But you didn't get it here at this hospital.

Me: No, I got it at the private office where I work.

Nurse: That sticker is unacceptable. You have to get a sticker from here.

Me: OK, give me a sticker.

Nurse: But you need a flu shot from here to get the sticker. Your sticker is unacceptable. So you need a flu shot today.

Me: First, I'm not getting another flu shot, that's crazy. Second, my sticker is much better than yours. All your sticker says is "FLU 16" and nothing else. Mine has the lot number, expiration date, and all sorts of information. Third, the only reason I'm in the hospital is to get Splenda for my coffee.

Nurse, *confused*: Well, if you're an employee here, then we should have a record of you getting the flu shot.

(*Nurse goes to computer and looks me up.*)

Nurse: It says here that you didn't get a flu shot.

Me: That's because I didn't get it in this hospital system. By that logic, I've never gotten any vaccines ever because I wasn't born at this hospital.

Nurse: I guess that's true.

Me: Great. Give me a sticker and let me get my Splenda!

After a fantastic day in the OR and the office . . .

Me: I always feel a bit manic after surgery goes really well. It makes me really happy, and I like to do stuff afterward.

Brother: So what did you do?

Me: I went to Home Depot with a friend. He had to get some painting supplies, and I bought a headlight.

Brother: You bought a headlight?

Me: Yeah. It's pretty sweet, 285 lumens, adjustable brightness and focus. Only twenty bucks!

Brother: But what happened to your old headlight?

Me: Eh. It stopped working. Also I lost it.

Brother: Wait, you bought a headlight for your car, right?

Me: No. I bought a headlight for my head.

Brother: Ohhh. I thought you were talking about your car.

Me: Nah, it's for when I have to go drain peritonsillar abscesses and whatnot.

Brother: You're an idiot.

Me: Manic!

Seeing patients in my clinic

Me: It says here you're here for your sinuses. What's going on?

Patient: I've been having this on-and-off sinus issue this past year ever since I moved up here from New Mexico. Bad nasal congestion and drip, and my eyes are itchy and watery.

Me: All right. Do you have allergies?

(*Long pause.*)

Patient: Well, I don't like it when things die.

Me: Um. I don't like it when things die either. But are you allergic to anything?

Patient: Yeah, like dead things.

(*Long pause.*)

Me: You're allergic to dead things?

Patient: Yeah, you know what I'm talking about, right?

Me: I have no idea what you're talking about.

Patient: You know, like dead things! They get all gunky and stuff.

Me: Oh, you mean, like mold, for instance? You're allergic to mold?

Patient: Yeah, but like dead mold. I might be allergic to other dead things too.

Me: You know what, it doesn't matter anymore. Let me take a look at you, and we'll send you to an allergist.

Called from ER

ER attending: I have kind of a weird question for you.

Me: I love weird questions! What do you got?

ER attending: I have a guy here who had sinus surgery yesterday in California, and he got on a flight today. He has some packing in his nose, and he wants it removed. We wanted to check with you.

Me: That's crazy. Who told him to get on a plane? Why is he here?

ER attending: He's like twenty-one years old, and he says he wants to party, but the packing is in the way.

Me: That's stupid. So tell him he's an idiot. And if you don't want to tell him that, you can say that I called him an idiot. Tell him he can go back to California to his surgeon to get that packing removed.

ER attending, *laughing*: He bought a one-way ticket.

Me: That's not my problem. I'm not getting involved in this nonsense. I mean, you know this is ridiculous, right?

ER attending: I do. Just want to make sure it's OK for him to have the packing in for a few more days. He's already on antibiotics.

Me: Great.

ER attending: Can we send him to your clinic?

Me: You can, but I'm going to tell them not to touch the guy. I don't know what type of surgery they did in California. I mean, what if we take out the packing and he has a massive bleed in the clinic and dies? Granted, that's a worst-case

Discontinue Leeches!!
And Other Stories from an ENT's Training

scenario, but nevertheless. If he really wants the packing out, he needs to call his surgeon and have him arrange for follow-up over here. I can't imagine that guy's gonna be very happy.

ER attending: Gotcha. Just wanted to check with you that it's all right to send him out.

Me: Not a problem. Happy to help.

Called for epistaxis in the middle of the night

Me, *to nurse*: I was wondering if you could help me out. I'm still figuring out where all your supplies are, and I need to pack this guy's nose. Do you have like an epistaxis kit or somewhere where you keep those supplies?

Nurse: Oh, we have an ENT cart.

Me: That sounds good. Should have what I need.

(*Nurse rolls over a cart with five drawers that's labeled "ENT." All five drawers are filled with four-by-four gauze pads.*)

Me: What am I supposed to do with this?

Nurse: That's the ENT cart. See, it says it right there.

Me: Sure that's what it says. But it's filled with four-by-fours.

Nurse: Well, this is our ENT cart.

Me: Well, you can label it whatever you want. I could label it a code cart, but do you want to try to resuscitate a dying person with four-by-fours?

Nurse: I guess you have a point.

Me: And I guess I'll figure something else out.

Ordering antibiotics for a patient. Get a page from pharmacy.

Pharmacist: You're taking care of Mr. Smith and ordered ceftriaxone?

Me: That's right.

Pharmacist: Why did you order ceftriaxone though?

Me: Well, the patient has a neck abscess. We cultured it, and it's sensitive to ceftriaxone.

Pharmacist: Well, you need an Infectious Disease consult to order ceftriaxone. We need their approval to dispense it.

Me: That seems excessive. Is there anything else I can order based on the sensitivities that doesn't need ID approval?

(*Pharmacist puts me on hold.*)

Pharmacist: Nope, everything needs ID approval. So it's three o'clock, it shouldn't be hard to get an ID consult.

Me: But what I'm telling you is that I don't need an ID consult. I know the source, I know the bacteria, and I know the sensitivities. What more are they going to tell me?

Pharmacist: Well, it's hospital policy.

Me: Well, that's stupid. I guarantee if I call the ID people, they're going to laugh at me.

(Call the ID resident and explain the situation to him.)

ID resident: But why do you need a consult?

Me: I don't. I just need your attending to say it's all right for me to give the antibiotic.

Attending in background: Whatever, it's fine. I've fucking had it with the Pharmacy at this hospital. What a waste of time.

ID resident: He says that's fine.

Me: No, I got the gist of it. Thanks!

(Call Pharmacy back with the attending's name.)

Pharmacist: So what did they say?

Me: You don't want to know. Can you just dispense this drug, please?

Seeing patients in clinic

Me: What brings you in here today?

Patient: I had a bit of a tickle in the back of my throat last week and a slight cough. The next day it turned into a bit of a runny nose.

Me: OK. Sounds like you had a cold. Did you take anything for it?

Patient: I went to the walk-in clinic, and they gave me a Z-pack. I also took Zyrtec, Benadryl, Afrin, and started Flonase.

(*Long pause.*)

Me: Um. You took those all at the same time?

Patient: Yeah, I figured I'd get a real handle on it. More is better, you know?

Me: Not always. How do you feel?

Patient: Well, my nose is really, really dry now.

Me: Yeah, I can imagine.

Patient: So what do I do?

Me: Stop all those medications. Rinse your nose out a couple of times a day with saline.

Patient: That's all? Don't I need antibiotics?

Me: Nope.

Patient: Then why did I come here?

Me: I don't know. But have a good day!

Introducing myself to a patient

Me: My name is Dr. Patel. I don't know if I met you the last time you were here.

Patient: You didn't because I'd remember that name. Amit.

Me: Oh. Why exactly?

Patient: I know five or six people named Amit. The name always makes me hungry.

Me: What now?

Patient: I love Indian food. All the spices!

Me: Oh. Interesting that my name in particular would do that.

Patient: You know what my favorite curry is? Palak Paneer.

Me: It is a good one.

Patient: I love it so much! Even though I try to avoid dairy products as much as possible.

Me: Well, they have pills for lactose intolerance these days.

Patient: No, I avoid it because I like to keep vegan.

Me: Oh well, they have pills for that too.

Patient, *laughs*: I'm not a very good vegan, am I?

Me: Doesn't sound like it.

A Nested Story a la 1001 Arabian Nights

(Talking with my cousin about a year ago when I was a chief resident)

Cousin: I really like your Facebook posts. But a lot of them revolve around something silly a patient says or something ridiculous interaction with hospital staff. I want one where you look silly.

Me: Well, there are enough of those. Here's one . . .

(*Taking the stairs between floors at the VA somewhere during my third year.*)

Chief resident: I notice you always check the doorknob on the other side of the door by turning it whenever you walk through. Why do you do that?

Me: Well, I'm checking if it will lock on me in case I need to get back through that door.

Chief: When did you start to do that?

Me: Well, let me tell you a story . . .

(*Taking overnight call as an intern during my first month of residency and have to get to the next floor up to do a postop check. Thinking I'll be clever, I decide to take the stairs so I don't look like a lazy person who takes the elevator up one floor. I find myself locked in the stairwell with no egress, so I call one of the nurses' stations.*)

Nurse: Who is this?

Me: My name's Amit Patel. I'm one of the surgical interns, and I'm locked in the stairwell.

Nurse, *laughing*: How did you do that?

Me: Well, I walked into the stairwell, and all the doors are locked. I tried going all the way down to the ground floor, but that door is locked too. So I'm stuck. Can you let me back in?

Nurse, *still laughing*: Hold on, some people gotta hear about this.

(*I hear the nurse telling other people at the station and general laughter.*)

Nurse, *still laughing*: Well, we're on break at the moment. Is this an emergency?

Me: Technically, no, but I do have work to do.

Nurse, *still laughing*: Someone will be by.

(*Ten minutes later, the nurse comes to let me back in.*)

Nurse, *still laughing*: Well, welcome to the hospital. Hope you learned something.

Me: I did. Thanks.

(*Back to talking to my chief during my third year.*)

Me: So that's why I always check the door.

Chief: You're an idiot.

Me: But an idiot who always has an escape plan!

(*Back to talking to my cousin while I was a chief.*)

Me: So that's one story of how I looked silly.

Cousin: Yeah, that does take you down a couple of notches.

Me: Thanks!

Called to drain an ear abscess on a young Italian girl

Me: So essentially, I have to make a small cut in the area of the swelling and release all the fluid.

Patient: Is it going to hurt?

Me: I'll numb it up as best as possible, but it may not take away all the pain, maybe just get it down to a dull roar.

Patient: What does this mean, a dull roar?

Me: Oh sorry, it means that there will be less pain but not gone completely.

Patient: Oh good, so this is how you say an idiom?

Me: Exactly.

Patient: I've learned something then.

(*Numb the ear up and make a small stab incision. Patient begins to sing in Italian.*)

Me: Are you doing all right? Not in too much pain?

Patient: No. I'm all right.

(*Press on the ear to get the infected fluid to come out. Patient begins to swear in Italian.*)

Patient: Sporca puttana! Pezzo di merda!

Me, *as I continue to work*: What exactly are you saying there?

Patient: Oh, I'm sorry, it's like a lot of bad words. Sorry, this is how I calm myself down. Singing and swearing.

Me: No, I got that, but what does it mean?

Patient: Oh, *puttana* is like "whore." Or like "slut," this is better. And *sporca*, I'm not sure, maybe "dirty"? And *merda*, well . . . you know merda.

Me: Yeah, I know merda. It sounds a lot better in Italian than English.

Patient: Well, of course, it does!

Me: Now I've learned something then. And no worries, I swear all the time to calm myself down.

Patient: Good.

Seeing patients in the office

Me: What brings you in today?

Patient: I got a cortisone injection, and my voice didn't get better. It happened like ten months ago. Then the voice got better. Then it got worse. Then I got another cortisone injection, and my voice didn't get better.

Me: OK. Hold on. Why don't you tell me what was going on with your voice before ten months ago?

Patient: What's there to tell? I got the injection, and it didn't get better.

Me: But what was wrong with your voice? Why did you get an injection? Was it normal? Was it rough? Was it weak? Did it get worse all of a sudden, or was it gradual?

Patient: But that's your job to find out.

(*Take a deep breath to calm myself.*)

Me: I can't find out if you don't tell me.

Patient: But I don't think I should have to tell you. You should find it out.

Me: Let me get my attending. He's going to want to hear this.

(*Go get the attending and tell him the story. Attending is incredulous. We go to see the patient.*)

Attending, *to patient*: What's wrong with your voice?

Patient: Like I told your fellow, I got the injection, and my voice didn't get better.

(*Patient proceeds to tell my attending the same things he told me.*)

Patient: Well, if you're not going to help me, then what should I do?

Attending: You won't let us help you though. We're asking very simple questions, and you're not giving us any answers. How can we figure anything out if you won't tell us anything?

Patient: Well, I'm going to go then.

(*Patient leaves.*)

Attending: That was unbelievable. I can't fucking stand crazy people. I swear to God, I can't. I'm too old for this shit. People are the worst.

Me: Yeah, that guy was nuts. So what should we do?

Attending: He can come back if he wants, but I'm not going to see him. He's your personal patient.

Me: Great!

Start to get a number of strange pages over the weekend. I call the paging operator to find out what's going on.

Me: I've been getting a number of gibberish pages to my cell. Is there anything going on with the pager system?

Operator: No, it must be your pager. We haven't received any complaints.

Me: OK.

(*Weird pages continue, so I call the operator back.*)

Me: So this is still happening.

Operator: Yeah, we've gotten a number of complaints now.

Me: How long before this is resolved? Because it seems like someone is trying to page me for an emergency, and I have no way of calling them back.

Operator: You'll just have to be patient.

Me: OK.

(*Weird pages continue, and another call is placed.*)

Me: This is getting ridiculous. And if it's the entire system, then it's a huge issue.

Operator: Well, if it really is an emergency, whoever is paging you can call me, and I can put them in touch with you.

Me: Have you considered that whoever is paging me might not know to do that?

Operator: I know you're frustrated, but you have to realize I can't do anything without my supervisor. She needs to approve anything I do.

Me: You should call your supervisor then!

Operator: She hasn't called back.

Me: Wait, how are you trying to get in touch with her?

Operator: I paged her.

(*Long pause.*)

Me: You paged her. Is she on the same paging system?

(*Long pause.*)

Operator: Yes.

Me: Then tell me how she's supposed to get the message to call you if the paging system is down?

Operator: Oh. I guess I'll call her.

Me: You need to fix this. I'm sure whoever is trying to call me is getting really angry, and when I do get in touch with them, they will scream at me and essentially compare me to Dr. Josef Mengele. I don't need that right now.

(*Long pause.*)

Operator: Sir, I'm sorry, we don't have a Dr. Mengele on staff here.

Me: Well, let's hope not. You know what, never mind. This is my cell phone number. Just call me when this is taken care of.

Seeing patients in the office

Me: What brings you in here today?

Patient: I had a tonsillitis a couple of weeks ago. Really bad sore throat, no cough, and there was all this white stuff on my tonsils. I saw my primary care doctor. She did a throat culture, and it showed strep.

Me: OK. Did you take antibiotics?

Patient: Yes. She gave me amoxicillin, and it got better a week ago.

Me: So what brings you in here today?

Patient: Well, she's just a primary care doctor. You're a throat specialist, and I really need my throat to be better. I'm in marketing, so I really need my throat to be better.

Me: Oh, I thought you said your throat did get better. Did something change?

Patient: Not really, but I think since the infection, one of my tonsils is microscopically bigger than the other.

(*Pause.*)

Me: Microscopically?

Patient: I have one of those curved mirrors, you know, for shaving? And I've been really vigilant about looking at my tonsils since the infection. And if I turn my head to the left, the right one looks microscopically bigger than the left.

Me: All right.

(Examine patient. Everything, including tonsils, is normal.)

Me: Everything looks fine.

Patient: Are you absolutely sure?

Me: Yes, no sign of an infection, tonsils are normal and symmetric, everything looks great.

Patient: Shouldn't you take a throat culture though? To make sure the infection is gone?

Me: No reason to do that. There's nothing to indicate an infection, and if you got better on the antibiotics, it likely means the infection is gone.

Patient: Are you sure there's nothing wrong with me?

Me: I don't understand. Do you want something to be wrong with you?

Patient: No, it's just that I'm at the doctor's office.

Me: And I just gave you a clean bill of health. Go and enjoy your day!

Patient, *uncertainly*: OK . . .

(*Patient leaves. A couple of minutes later, I hear a big commotion followed by silence. I walk out to the secretary.*)

Me: What happened?

Secretary: Your last patient didn't want to pay for the visit.

Me: Why not?

Secretary: Did you tell him there was nothing was wrong with him?

Me: Yes . . . because there was nothing wrong with him.

Secretary: He didn't want to pay unless there was something wrong because he's paying out of pocket because we're not in his insurance network.

Me: Well, he was hot to trot for a specialist's opinion, not my fault he disagreed. Jeez, he really should've just gone back to his primary care doctor!

In Chicago for Oral Boards, get on elevator at hotel. Everyone else is wearing a badge that says "Examiner."

Examiner 1, *looks at me*: Oh, boy, surrounded by examiners!

Me: Looks that way.

Examiner 2: Maybe we should all start cackling evilly.

Examiner 3, 4, and 5: Mwahaha!

(*Elevator arrives at my floor.*)

Me, *as dryly as possible*: Thanks, guys.

Seeing a patient in the office

Me: So what it sounds like is going on is adductor spasmodic dysphonia. Essentially, your vocal cords are squeezing together inappropriately when you're talking.

Patient: Oh wow, really?

Me: Yes. Pretty uncommon altogether, but it is treatable with Botox injections to weaken those muscles so your voice isn't so strained.

Patient: Oh, I don't want any injections or anything like that. What else can we do?

Me: Sometimes neurologists can prescribe different oral medications, but they tend to be sedating. And speech therapy doesn't really help with this.

Patient: Well, I don't want to take medication either. Listen, I've noticed when I talk in an accent, especially an Irish accent, my voice is pretty much normal.

Me: Yeah, that's a known phenomenon. It's a sort of sensory trick to fool your brain from firing these inappropriate signals to the larynx.

Patient: Well, what about that?

Me: What about what?

Patient: What if I just talk in an accent all the time?

Me: Um . . .

Patient: I wouldn't need any shots or medications.

Discontinue Leeches!!
And Other Stories from an ENT's Training

Me: Well . . . I guess. Honestly the treatment is based around the symptoms. If you don't think it's interfering with your life, you don't need to do anything if you don't want. And if you want to talk in an accent all the time, that's up to you.

Patient: Great, I love my Irish accent. I'll come back if I want anything else. Thanks!

(Sometimes people are incredible.)

Seeing patients in the office

Me: So how are you feeling today?

Patient: Pretty good, but I'm kinda nervous about this Botox injection.

Me: Well, we'll try to diffuse the situation with some idle conversation.

Patient: OK.

Me: It's a beautiful day outside! How are you going to spend it?

Patient: Well, just walked through Central Park, and I saw all the people trying to get tans. I figured I'd go there a reread one of my favorite books.

Me: That sounds wonderful. What are you going to be reading?

Patient: Oh, I'm rereading the *Harry Potter* series. I'm on the third one.

Me: *The Prisoner of Azkaban!* That's actually my favorite.

Patient: Mine too!

(*Attending walks in.*)

Attending: Are you ready to do this?

Patient: Well, I was about as nervous as Harry Potter before the first Triwizard task, but this conversation with your fellow has really helped out.

Attending: What the hell are you talking about?

Me: Well, the first task was the one with the dragons. So she's doing pretty well!

Attending: All right, whatever works.

Tales from the clinic—patient with a seroma of her ear who also reeks of alcohol

Me: It looks like this fluid collection has come back even after they aspirated it twice.

Patient: That's right.

Me: Well, at this point, you have two options. We can try putting a needle in and sucking out the fluid again. I don't recommend that because it's been tried twice and hasn't worked. The other option is to make a small incision, drain the fluid out, and put a compressive dressing on it so the fluid can't recollect.

Patient: Dressing? I don't want no dressing on my ear.

Me: You'd need the dressing. Otherwise, there's no point.

Patient: What color is the dressing going to be?

Me: Excuse me?

Patient: It's going to be white, isn't it! Look at my skin! Do I look white to you? Are you going to give me a sharpie to color it in?

Me: Actually, the dressing is yellow.

Patient: Fucking white people, they don't ever help us out. How big?

Me: How big is the dressing? Big enough to cover the area of swelling.

Patient: No, no, no! I can't have no dressing on my ear! I got dates this weekend! What if someone wants to put their tongue or something else sweet in my ear?

Me: Oh god.

(*At this point, the patient pulls a bottle of malt liquor out of her purse and starts drinking it.*)

Me: You can't drink that in here.

Patient: So you can put that needle in, 'cause I'm not having a dressing.

Me: You need to go to the ER to dry out. Then we can talk about what to do to your ear.

Talking to My Attending

Me: So one of the PAs just called me. Our patient just got back from the CT scanner. He's got multiple PEs.

Attending: Hm. OK, good thing we got that scan.

Me: I told them to start a heparin drip.

Attending: Good work. I just don't know what we're going to do with this guy. First, he delays his own care by disappearing for two years to get herbal therapy. Then his disease is so extensive that the operation took twice as long as it should have. Now this.

Me: Yeah, you don't have luck with these laryngectomies, do you?

Attending: For real. I mean, my last one spent two months in the hospital. Maybe I should get rid of those earrings.

Me: What now? Earrings?

Attending: It occurred to me this morning that I was wearing the same set of earrings for both of those operations. They are clearly bad luck. So they have to go.

Me: I know exactly what you mean. I once got rid of a pair of socks because they caused a number of airway disasters.

Attending: I mean, I know scientifically that superstition doesn't make sense, but it's the truth! The universe is always watching what we do.

Me: I agree 100 percent.

Attending: It's a shame, they were a nice pair of earrings.

Tales from clinic. Seeing a ninety-year-old lady.

Me: Hi my name is Dr. Patel. I see you were sent here for . . . (*check referral*) . . . syphilis. Hm.

Patient: That's right. Every time I eat, stuff comes out my nose. And I can't hear!

Me: OK. Let's take a look.

(*Patient opens her mouth and has a hole in her hard palate.*)

Me: You have a hole in the roof of your mouth. Syphilis can do that. So when you try to swallow, instead of food going down into the esophagus, it comes out of your nose.

Patient: Oh! You're such a nice handsome young doctor. I like your hair.

Me: Thank you. Actually, I just bought some new shampoo the other day.

Patient: I could do things to you.

Me: Excuse me?

Patient: You heard me. I could do things to you.

Me: Let's focus on your problems first, shall we?

Patient: If you say so.

Seeing a patient with my attending

Attending: This is one of my earliest patients from when I was still doing some general ENT. I follow her for her ears.

Me: Wow, I bet you're glad you're not doing that any longer.

Attending: She's a sweet lady. Actually, she has a pretty interesting tympanic membrane and middle ear exam. She's in the other room. Why don't you take a look and tell me what you think?

(Go into the next room and examine patient. Both ears are PACKED with wax. Spend twenty minutes cleaning them out. Eardrums are completely normal. I go out and find my attending.)

Attending: So what did you think?

Me: Um, her ears are normal. I think you sent me in there just to clean out her ears.

Attending, *laughing*: Pretty much, yup.

Me: Underhanded technique! You know you could have just told me to clean out her ears. You're my attending and are allowed to do that.

Attending: But that's not as fun, is it?

Me: Yeah, you're right.

Show up to my attending's office hours after being up all night in the OR with a patient

Me: Do you have any recommendations for coffee?

Attending: What type of coffee? You want a pick-me-up or jet fuel?

Me: Jet fuel. I was in the OR all night with a disaster patient.

Attending: There's a place right a couple of blocks down on the right-hand side. Nice Brazilian place. Super strong coffee. In fact, pick me up some while you're there.

Me: OK.

(I leave and am waiting for the elevator. The attending runs up to me.)

Me: What's up?

Attending: I forgot to give you the little rewards card. Why don't you get coffee for the staff as well, and make sure they stamp the heck out of this thing?

Me: Quick question, would you ever ask a resident to do this?

Attending: No way! The ACGME would be all over me if I abused a resident like that. But you're a fellow. I can do whatever I want to you 'cause you signed up for this.

Me: Perfect.

Seeing patients in the office. Patient had been seen six years ago for a benign growth in his salivary gland.

Me: What brings you in here today?

Patient: I've had this lump under my neck for the past six years. I'm here to have it taken out.

Me: Um. OK. It's been getting bigger?

Patient: Listen, no offense to you, I didn't come here to talk to you. I came here to see your attending. I haven't eaten anything since last night so I could have surgery today.

Me: I'm going to take a little bit of offense. But whatever. I am going to tell you that you're not having surgery today. That's not how it works.

Patient: We'll see what your boss has to say about that.

(Go to talk to attending.)

Attending: Yeah, so we did an entire workup six years ago, and he has a benign tumor. He wanted to watch it then, and then I never heard from him again. Then he called me this weekend through my answering service in a panic from Massachusetts because he felt that it had gotten bigger. He wanted me to meet him at the emergency room. I told him he could go to the emergency room, but there was no chance in hell of me meeting him there.

Me: Well, he thinks he's having surgery today. He's been NPO since midnight.

Attending: That's stupid.

Me: Oh, I know.

(Go to see patient.)

Attending: I realize you want surgery, but it's something that has to be scheduled. You have some medical problems and need clearance. This is not an emergency and does not need to be done right away. But we can do it in a couple of weeks.

Patient: That's ridiculous. I work in investment banking, and we move a lot quicker than that!

Attending, *annoyed*: Then have an investment banker take this thing out. Don't involve me with it.

Patient: But I'm ready today! I haven't had anything to eat since last night.

Attending, *more annoyed*: That's ridiculous. Who told you to do that? Like I said, we'll be able to do it in a couple of weeks.

Patient: But I'll be at a wedding then.

Attending, *getting angry*: So either this is something urgent for you or it isn't. You can't have it both ways.

Patient: Well, what about the surgery? Tell me about that.

Attending: We put you to sleep, put a breathing tube in, make an incision in your neck, and remove the gland. We have some nerves to identify and avoid—

Patient, *interrupting*: Wait, it's a real surgery?

Attending, *getting even angrier*: I only do real surgery. I don't do fake surgery.

Patient: But from what I read on the Internet, it should only take ten minutes.

(*Long pause.*)

Attending: You know what, I have a feeling it isn't going to work out with us. I'm not getting involved in doing your surgery. It's not an emergency, and you can go see someone else, and I'll forward all your records to them. But I can't deal with you anymore.

(*Attending walks out of the room.*)

Patient: What happened?

Me: We're all done here.

Patient: Should I come back?

Me: Nope. Find another ENT, and we'll send them your records. But don't bother coming back.

Starting the day in clinic

Me: This sheet says it's a follow-up patient. Did we pull the chart?

Secretary: There are no more charts.

Me: What do you mean no more charts? How am I supposed to get her old records and see why she was here?

Secretary: I don't know. Let me call the clinic manager.

(*Clinic manager comes in.*)

Clinic manager: Yeah, so as of last week, we're not creating charts for patients anymore. We're in the process of transitioning to electronic medical records.

Me: Sure, but what about patients that came here while we still had paper records?

Clinic manager: Those charts are offsite being scanned into a database where you can access the images from.

Me: I don't have access to that.

Clinic manager: None of the doctors have access to it. It's not set up yet.

Me: But that's stupid. We have patients here that have been seen before, and I can't get any of their records. So what am I supposed to do? Tell patients that we don't have access to their records and start over from the beginning? That's ridiculous.

Clinic manager: Yeah, I can understand your frustration. Unfortunately, it was a poorly thought-up and executed plan.

Me: That's not my problem though. So here's what we're going to do. Unless the patient says it's an absolute emergency, I'm refusing to see any follow-up patients that we don't have access to their records until you can figure out a way of getting those records back here. They can be rescheduled to another day. And you can explain to them why exactly they're not being seen today. I don't want to have anything to do with that.

Clinic manager: You want me to explain?

Me: Yes, because this was an administrative decision, and no doctor was involved in it. I mean, how would you feel if you showed up to your doctor's office and they told you they'd essentially lost all of your records?

Clinic manager: I'd be pretty upset. Hmmm, I guess I didn't think of it that way.

Me: Doesn't sound like anyone thought it through.

Prepping to do a tracheostomy

Circulator: What's your name?

Me: My name's Amit Patel.

Circulator: And you're from what service? General Surgery?

Me: ENT.

Circulator: But what are you, the medical student?

Me: No, the attending.

Circulator: But you look like you're twelve years old.

Me: Really? Even with a beard? And some gray hairs?

Circulator: You could have just borrowed those from your father.

Me: You know, the few times I've been told I look too young to be an attending is when I have a beard. When I shave my beard and I actually look like I'm twelve years old, nobody bats an eye.

(*Anesthesia attending walks in, and we exchange introductions. Then she looks at me with a very puzzled expression.*)

Me: You look worried about something.

Anesthesiologist: Your ID tag says that you're a volunteer.

Me: Oh, that's the ID tag for the other hospital I go to. I don't have malpractice insurance there, so the best title they can give me is volunteer.

(*I flip to my other ID and show her the attending title.*)

Anesthesiologist: Oh, that's funny. Here I thought for a second the hospital administrators had found another way to save money by just finding volunteers off the street to do trachs for them.

Me: Well, I wouldn't put it past them.

SITTING AT NURSES' STATION WRITING NOTES ON PATIENTS

Nurse, *yelling into phone*: Folake Chukwu! Folake Chukwu!

Phone: You have logged in as Felicia Christian. Is this correct?

Nurse: No Folake Chukwu!

Phone: You have logged in as Felicia Christian. Is this correct?

Nurse, *hangs up phone*: This thing is so stupid!

Me: What are you trying to do?

Nurse: Oh, the hospital decided to take away the overhead paging system from the nurses' station, and they made us put this app on our phone so we could get in touch with one another.

Me: Sounds like it doesn't work very well with Nigerian names.

Nurse: It doesn't work well with any names. So now we just yell down the hallway.

Me: Classic.

Nurse: Why are you asking? You want one of these?

Me: No way, I'm just curious why you were yelling. The less people that can get in touch with me, the better.

Seeing patients in the office; chief complaint, "Breathing is good through the nose."

Me: This is an odd chief complaint. Have we seen this patient before? Maybe we gave him some allergy medication or did surgery on him a long time ago?

(*Nurse looks through the old charts.*)

Nurse: No, he's a brand-new patient.

(*Go to see patient.*)

Me: What seems to be the problem?

Patient: I want my nose checked out. My breathing is good through my nose.

Me: I don't really understand. Did something happen to your nose?

Patient: It's like this. I was out clubbing a couple of months ago and got into a fight, and someone broke my nose. It all healed up, but then I couldn't breathe through the right side. Then a couple of weeks ago, I was out clubbing again and I got into a fight and I got punched in the nose again. It all healed up, and now my breathing is better.

Me: Where were you out clubbing where you were getting into so many fights?

Patient: Hoboken.

Me: Sure, makes sense. Well, let's take a look.

(*Scope patient with attending—nasal septum looks like it's been fractured many times but is remarkably midline.*)

Attending: You should stop getting punched in the nose.

Patient: I try, but you know how it is.

Attending: No, I don't know.

(*Patient leaves happy.*)

Attending: That guy was pretty stupid. Although, this reminds me of the case study from a long time ago where some guy in Canada fixed his own septum by sticking his finger in his nose and pushing the septum to the midline every day for a year. They called it digital auto-septoplasty.

Me: Really? That was published?

Attending: Yeah, look it up.

(*Look up reference.*)

Me: Jeez, that was nearly thirty years ago, and you remember that?

Attending: There's a part of my brain that registers ridiculous stuff.

Me: Awesome.

Seeing patients in the office

Patient: So I was with my friend Michael Keaton, the actor, and we were talking for a while. And my voice was getting bad! So Michael leans over to me and asks me if I'm sick. And I say no, so he's like, "Dude, you better get that shit checked out. It could be something bad."

Attending: Fair enough.

(*Examine the patient and find his vocal cords are thin.*)

Attending: So nothing dangerous is going on. Your vocal cords are a bit thin from aging, and you have to put a bit more effort in to talk, so your voice gets worse more easily.

Patient: Phew, so all this is because I'm old as fuck? I'm gonna go tell Michael he's full of shit.

Attending: Well, he was concerned about you!

Patient: I'm just kidding. Lemme ask you something. I went to a hockey game at Chelsea Piers at two in the fucking morning the other day, screamed my head off, and lo and behold, my voice was great the next day. Why is that?

Attending: That's because your vocal cords are thin, so when you scream, you cause a little bit of swelling. They plump up, and you sound better.

Patient: That's really amazing. So oral sex would be a good thing for me?

(*Silence.*)

Attending: Well . . . no comment.

Patient: Great, I gotcha. Well, thanks for everything.

(*Patient leaves.*)

Me: So we just got a consult from Batman.

Attending: Yeah, that guy was a real trip. Still trying to figure out that oral sex thing though.

Me: Well, he's obviously doing something wrong.

Attending: Seemingly.

Last call of fellowship, pager goes off at 3:00 AM.

Me: Hi, it's ENT, what's up?

ICU resident: Oh, hey, I paged you four hours ago!

Me: Hm. Well, that's probably going to be an issue. Sorry about that, my pager literally just went off. What's going on?

ICU resident: Well, nothing now, but before, one of the patients I think one of your PAs had packed yesterday had some bleeding from his nose around the packing.

Me: All right.

ICU resident: But it stopped after about an hour. He's not tachycardic, hemoglobin is stable. It's probably because his platelets are five, so we transfused him.

Me: Sounds fantastic.

ICU resident: Well, we just wanted your recommendations on what to do.

Me: Well, I think you've done a great job. No amount of packing will stop someone that wants to bleed. And anyway, as you know, all bleeding eventually stops.

ICU resident: Wow, did you just make that up?

Me: Nope, that's a universal truth in medicine. Anyway, as long as you're happy.

ICU resident: I'm not. All I want to do is rheumatology, and I'm stuck in the ICU.

Me: Well, that sucks. Good luck!

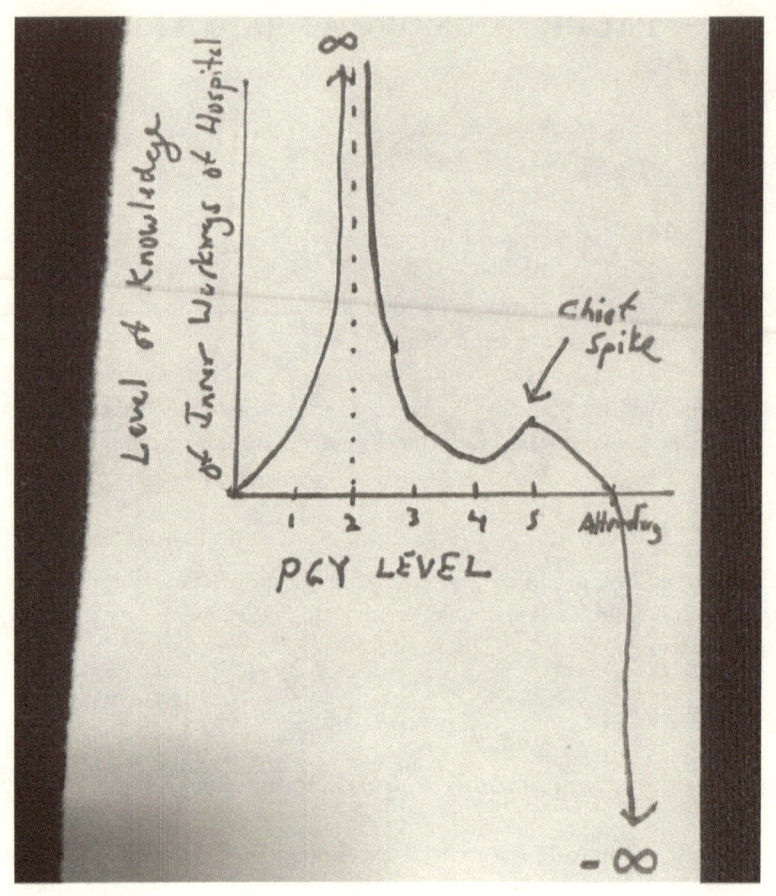

ATTENDING

Trying to get credentialed, but first, I have to meet with the chairman of surgery. Call the office to make an appointment.

Secretary: Department of Surgery.

Me: Hi, my name's Amit Patel. I'm going to be joining the local ENT practice, and I'm trying to get credentialed at the hospital—

Secretary, *cutting me off*: OK, well this is the Department of General Surgery. We have nothing to do with credentialing.

Me: Um—

Secretary, *talking over me*: That is not what I do. In fact, this is the Chairman's Office, and I take care of him and his schedule.

Me: Yes, but—

Secretary: You need to be talking to Mrs. Jones down in credentialing. I don't know who you are.

Me: Uh—

Secretary: I didn't get any e-mails from her regarding you. If you really want to get credentialed, you should be talking to her and not me. This is the Department of Surgery.

(*Period of silence.*)

Me: Great, I really appreciate that information. So I got an e-mail from Mrs. Jones this morning to call you to make an appointment with the chairman of Surgery specifically for credentialing.

(*Long pause.*)

Secretary: Oh. Well, then I'm exactly whom you need to be talking to. Why didn't you say that before? How's Monday at ten?

(Everybody fiercely guards their own little fiefdom in a hospital.)

END OF A DAY OF BILLING AND CODING TRAINING

Trainer: So how do you feel? Think you got it?

Me: I think so. If I overcode and bill, that's bad.

Trainer: Yes.

Me: If I undercode, that's bad too.

Trainer: Yes.

Me: But there's a good chance I'm going to overcode and undercode without realizing it.

Trainer: Yes. And we'll try to let you know if you're doing either.

Me: And the government is watching everything.

Trainer: Exactly. Sounds like you got the basics. Good luck starting!

Me: Thanks!

END OF THE FIRST DAY OF SEEING PATIENTS. ANOTHER DOCTOR IN THE PRACTICE COMES UP TO ME.

Doctor: So how did your first day go?

Me: Yeah, not bad. I feel like my head is spinning with this medical record system. It feels like I did so much more work than I actually accomplished today.

Doctor: Yeah, it's terrible. And don't worry, you're gonna feel like your head is spinning for at least the first three months. If you don't feel lost, you're doing something wrong.

Me: Oh perfect!

SEEING PATIENTS IN THE OFFICE. MEDICAL ASSISTANT COMES IN TO TELL ME ABOUT THE PATIENT.

Me: So what's this kiddo here for?

MA: He's been having some ear problems. Looks like mom saw a cyst in his ear canal.

Me: Hm. Any history of ear problems or surgeries?

MA: Not that I know of, but he did have some sort of surgery last year. A me-plasty?

Me: What's that now? An M-plasty? Like a scar revision?

MA: No, they said me-plasty.

Me: Um . . . maybe a meatoplasty?

MA: Yeah, that's it!

Me: Well, that's a type of ear surgery for sure.

MA, *looking puzzled*: Really? They said the urologist did it.

Me, *burst out laughing*: Oh, like a urethral meatoplasty! Never mind!

MA: I'm so confused.

Me: Don't worry about it, you've just been witness to one of those rare crossovers between urology and ENT. Doesn't happen often, but when it does, it's fantastic.

Seeing a very nice man with mental retardation who needs his ears cleaned

Me: Hello, sir, my name is Dr. Patel.

Patient, *eyes get very wide*: Are you GOD?

Me: Um . . . not that I know of.

Patient: You look like my priest! Are you God?

Me: Oh well, I hope he's a nice person. I'm not God.

Patient: If you're not God, then I'm not listening to you.

(He is accompanied by his caretaker, whom I look to for help.)

Caretaker: He's very religious. But you have to tell him you're God if you're gonna want to clean his ears. It's not right, but it's the only way he'll let you examine him.

Me: Mr. Smith, this is God! I need to look in your ears!

Patient: OK.

(*Clean his ears without any problems.*)

Me: You're all done!

Patient: Thank you, God!

Me: You're very welcome.

(Gotta do what you gotta do to take care of your patients.)

SEEING A PATIENT IN THE OFFICE FOR CHRONIC SORE THROAT

Patient: You have no idea! I take antibiotics, I take steroids, it gets better, and then it comes back! I just keep getting these tonsil infections.

Me: I'm sorry you're going through this. Anything else make it better or worse?

Patient: Well, I tried this old home remedy my grandmother used to give to my mother back in Guatemala. My mother mailed some to me, and I think it helped. I can look it up for you.

Me: That's all right.

Patient, *going through her phone*: No, hold on a second, you could give it to your other patients. Here it is.

(*Patient shows me her phone on which is written "TETRACICLINA."*)

Me, *after a long pause*: Tetracycline?

Patient: Yeah, I think it helped.

Me: That's an antibiotic though.

Patient: No, it's not! It's something my grandmother used to make for my mother. Now she made it for me.

Me: No, that's an antibiotic. I doubt your grandmother was making it.

Patient: Why would they tell me that then?

Me: Maybe you should call your grandmother. Any other symptoms?

New attending anxieties

Had to send my first patient to be admitted to the hospital today. Without going into specifics, I'd seen him a couple of days ago, started antibiotics, but his parents called today saying he wasn't getting better, and he definitely looked worse when I brought him to the office. But how do I admit a patient to the hospital from a private practice?

I have to call the pediatrician. But the pediatrician doesn't have admitting privileges at the hospital. OK, so I have to call the emergency room. But what's the number to the emergency room? Or the hospital for that matter? And how does it work in terms of the politics down here? Do the specialists admit their own patients or does a hospitalist? Is there a way of talking with the hospitalist before I send the patient there? I'm not on call this weekend, but should I round on this patient? The other partners have told me they round on all the patients in the practice who are admitted, no matter who initially saw or operated on them, but I feel like I'd ruin the weekend of the guy who's on call just by having him check a kid's ear. He'll probably end up questioning my clinical judgment asking why this kid even needed to go to the hospital. Wait, does this kid actually need to be admitted?

At this point, I'm chewing the inside of my cheek because that's what I do when I'm nervous/anxious. WTF, this would've been so easy at as a resident; just call the Peds ER and tell them you're sending a kiddo to the ER, call patient transport, and that's that! I'm paralyzed by my own lack of knowledge of the inner and outer workings of the regional health-care system, which, having a type A personality, leads me to question my own ability as a physician. I know this is quite ludicrous, but it is what it is.

Finally end up talking it over with another doctor in the practice, who helps me make some phone calls and is superunderstanding about everything. He assures me that within a short time, this will be second nature and I won't have to worry about it, but I don't feel reassured at all.

Prior to my first attending call

Partner: Dude, you're on call tomorrow. Are you nervous?

Me: Only about having to figure out where stuff is and that nonsense.

Partner: Oh, you'll be fine. Listen, man, call here is pretty light altogether. You have the occasional disaster, but it's pretty great. Nothing's gonna happen to you.

Me: Well, there you go. Why would you say that?

Partner, *catching my drift*: Oh, so you're one of those . . .

Me: A black cloud? Definitely.

Partner, *laughing*: Hm . . . maybe we made a mistake hiring you.

Me: You laugh now. Only time will tell.

Overheard at the Front Desk Through a Closed Door

Secretary: Ma'am, you're scheduled for a hearing test today. Do you not want it?

Lady, *clearly elderly, with a thick New Jersey accent*: A WHAT? WHAT DO I NEED?

Her son, *with equally thick accent*: MA! LISTEN TO ME! MA! YOU NEED THE HEARING TEST!

Secretary: You don't have to get it today, but we can reschedule it.

Lady: WELL, HOW LONG IS THAT GONNA TAKE? I AIN'T GOT ALL DAY. I JUST CAME HERE TO GET THE WAX OUT!

Secretary: Well, based on our schedule, it'll be about forty-five minutes or so.

Lady: FORTY-FIVE MINUTES? I AIN'T GOT THAT LONG! LISTEN, I'M NINETY-SIX GODDAMN YEARS OLD! IF I MAKE IT TO DINNER TONIGHT, I THINK I'M PRETTY LUCKY!

Son: MA! WE'VE BEEN OVER THIS! GET THE GODDAMN HEARING TEST! YA CAN'T UNDERSTAND ANYONE!

Lady: I DON'T WANT NO GODDAMN HEARING AIDS! I JUST WANT THE WAX OUT! I DON'T WANT TO LOOK LIKE I'M OLD!

Son: GODDAMN IT, MA! WE COME HERE EVERY MONTH TO GET YOUR EARS CLEANED. JUST GET THE HEARING TEST!

(*I turn to the other physician in the room.*)

Discontinue Leeches!! And Other Stories from an ENT's Training

Me: Is it usually like this?

Other doc: Every now and then.

Me: Maybe they can take the crackpot convention outside?

Other doc: Eh, the staff is used to it. Welcome to the practice!

Down to my last patient of the day and eager to leave. Trying to be as efficient as possible. I come in and shake the patient's hand.

Me: Hello, sir, how are you doing?

Patient: Terrible. My ear is killing me. It gets clogged with wax all the time.

Me, *putting on pair of gloves*: OK, well we'll have a look. Anything else bothering you? Drainage from the ears? Sore throat?

Patient: Nah, just the ear.

Me: OK, I'll take a look in just a second. Let me just log onto my computer.

(*Computer uses a fingerprint scanner to log on, which doesn't seem to be working.*)

Me, *wondering out loud*: Hm, it doesn't seem to be working.

(*Patient remains silent.*)

Me, *after several attempts*: You know, technology is supposed to make your life easier, but sometimes it really doesn't.

Patient: Um, that's a fingerprint scanner, right? Probably won't work if you have gloves on.

(*Long silence.*)

Discontinue Leeches!!
And Other Stories from an ENT's Training

Me, *looking at my gloved hands*: Well, shit, you're definitely right about that. Sorry, didn't mean to swear there.

(*Take off my gloves and log in.*)

Patient, *laughing*: Long week?

Me: You have no idea. Let's see about that ear, shall we?

Telling a Story About How My Dad's Snoring Kept Our Family Up During Vacations

Me: Well, he's much better now that he has the CPAP.

Cousin: Is that the only thing you can do? The CPAP?

(*Talk a bit about sleep surgery.*)

Cousin: So let me get this straight. My dad has sleep apnea. Your dad has sleep apnea. Your other uncles have all these sleep problems, and you're telling us all these wonderful things you can do, but all you do is take care of people that sing, which no one in this family can do? Is that what you're telling me?

(*Everyone starts laughing.*)

Me: Well, when you put it that way, yes.

Brother: No one's gonna top that.

On marketing one's self—talking with one of the medical assistants

MA: We really should get your name out there! Just so you can get referrals and more patients.

Me: Thanks, but I'm pretty sure our marketing department has that covered. They have a pretty good marketing team.

MA: Nah, but you need that local touch. Really get your name into the hospitals.

Me: Hm. What are you thinking?

MA: Well, I used to work in a private practice with one of the other docs who works here now. When he first started, I used to call the hospital and just overhead page him.

Me: What?

MA: Yeah, once or twice a day, I'd overhead page him whether or not he was there. That way, people heard his name and associated him with ENT.

Me: Yeah, but aren't you supposed to only overhead page in case of emergencies?

MA: Technically, yeah, but at least everyone in the hospital knew who he was.

Me: Um, thanks, but no. I'm pretty sure they were thinking, *Who the hell is this new doctor, and why is he getting paged to so many emergencies? He must really not know what he's doing!*

MA: You sure? OK.

Seeing patients in office

Me: Nice to meet you. Let me just turn off my phone.

(*Put phone in pocket without looking and then absentmindedly scratch the side of my face and put on a pair of gloves.*)

Me: What brings you in here today?

Patient, *grinning*: My ears are filled with wax.

Me: OK, you seem to be happy about that.

Patient: No, but you make me laugh.

Me: What?

Patient: Oh nothing.

Me: OK, that's weird, but let's take a look.

(*Clean out the patient's ears while he's laughing. Entire situation is strange.*)

Me: You're all done!

Patient, *still laughing*: Thanks, doc!

(*Patient leaves, and I walk out bewildered.*)

Medical assistant: You know you have a huge ink stain on your pants and down the side of your face, right?

Discontinue Leeches!!
And Other Stories from an ENT's Training

(*Look down at my hand, and sure enough, my pen had exploded. Look in a mirror, and there's a big ink stain on my face.*)

Me: Well, the laughing is making more sense. Too bad I don't have a change of pants.

Seeing patients in the office

Me: What brings you in here today?

Patient: I have pneumonia, and my stomach hurts.

Me: What? Pneumonia?

Patient: Yeah, I know it's because I smoke. I'm always coughing up a lot of mucus, and then I get these fevers and short of breath. But the antibiotics always make it better. I cough so much that my belly hurts.

Me: Ma'am, this is an ear, nose, and throat office. Do you have any issues with those?

Patient: No, I told you I have pneumonia.

Me: OK, that's a little outside my wheelhouse. Why didn't you see your primary care doctor?

Patient: 'Cause it takes six hours to be seen by them. It was easier to get an appointment with you. You're a doctor, so you can take care of me.

Me: I don't really treat pneumonias per se. Not my specialty.

Patient: You went to medical school, didn't you? You should be able to take care of everything.

Me: Maybe, but you wouldn't want to see me about, say, a foot issue.

Patient: Well, I'm not leaving here unless I get some antibiotics and pain medication.

(*And so on and so forth.*)

On building your patient base

Medical assistant: Mrs. Smith is here. She's very excited to see you.

Me: Have I seen her before?

MA: No, but you've seen her daughter.

Me: What's her daughter's name?

MA: I don't know, didn't ask.

Me: OK.

(*Go to see the patient.*)

Patient: Oh, Dr. Patel, do you remember me? I came here with my daughter back in September.

Me, *more ebullient than I otherwise am*: Of course, I remember you! How have you been? How is your daughter? I hope she's doing well.

Patient: Oh, my ears are bothering me. I think I have wax. You took such good care of my daughter when you took out her earwax, she was raving about it for days!

Me: OK, so you're here for earwax too?

Patient: Definitely. You know how it runs in families.

Me: Let's take a look.

(*Patient has a minimal amount of earwax, which I clean out.*)

Me: OK, all done!

Patient: Oh, that was wonderful! Listen, I know you're a new doctor, and I'm going to do you a favor. Every person I know that has earwax, I'm going to send your way. Because you're so young and need to build a practice. And I know a lot of people with earwax.

Me, *in my head*: NOOOOOOOOOOOOOOO!

Me, *out loud*: Well, I really appreciate that. Thank you so much!

(*Patient leaves, and MA comes in.*)

MA: So did you remember her?

Me: No idea who she was or who her daughter was. Oh well, she was happy.

SEEING A TWENTY-SOMETHING PATIENT FOR A RUNNY NOSE

Me: So it says here you're here for a runny nose.

Patient: No, that's stopped. But I need to stop them from happening.

Me: Oh OK, is this an ongoing issue?

Patient: No, this is the first time it's happened this year.

Me: Hm, did you have any other symptoms?

Patient: I had a bit of a cough, and my throat was kinda sore. Lasted for a few days and then went away. And this happened last year too!

Me: Any allergies? Fevers? Chills?

Patient: Nope.

Me: Well, it sounds like you had a cold. But let's take a look at you.

(*Examine the patient; everything is normal.*)

Me: Yeah, so it sounds like you had a cold, and you're over it.

Patient: But you need to cure me.

Me: Um . . . cure you of what?

Patient: I can't ever get a cold again.

Me: What?

Patient: I can't ever get a cold again. You have to do something.

Me: It was a cold, likely a virus that you picked up from somewhere, and your own immune system took care of it. They're very common. People get colds. It's the common cold!

Patient: Ugh, typical. You doctors are always trying to keep the real treatments away from us patients. I've been to three other doctors, and they've told me the same thing.

Me: OK, well, you can help prevent yourself from getting a cold by observing basic hygiene. Washing hands, avoiding people who do have colds, and whatnot. But it's not like you're never going to get a cold again.

Patient: No, you have a cure, and I know it. You're just holding out.

Me: I don't understand what you want from me. Believe me, if I had a cure for the common cold, I'd be a billionaire with a Nobel Prize.

Patient: You're all against me! So is that it?

Me: Yeah, that's it. Wash your hands!

Seeing a patient for something or the other in the office

Patient: Can I ask you a question?

Me: Sure, what's up?

Patient: I really like your watch.

Me: Not really a question, but thank you!

Patient: No, so my question is, and I don't mean to offend you in any way, and you don't have to answer, but . . . I've worked with a lot of Indian people and they all really love gold. Why is that?

Me, *laughing*: You're completely right, Indian people love gold. It's a way to show off wealth, and plus I think since they don't really trust the government, it's a way of putting your money into something somewhat tangible.

Patient: OK, that's why I noticed your watch. Because it's not gold.

Me: Well, I'm not like most Indian people. But I'm pretty sure I have a gold chain somewhere. Any health-related questions?

Patient: No, you've answered everything.

Me: Great.

Walk into exam room to find an older lady is doing a word find puzzle

Me: Hi, my name is Dr. Patel. What brings you in here today?

Patient: Just a second, I'm almost done.

Me: I see you like doing word finds. I'm a crossword puzzle person myself.

Patient: I used to do those, but you know, I find these are better for my mental health. Keeps my vision and attention sharp. Not like all the old fuddy-duddies in my building.

(*I glance at the chart; patient is eighty-seven years old.*)

Patient: You know, I was in my building the other day, and some person was trying to give me another tenant's mail. You know what I said to him?

Me: I don't know.

Patient: What do you think I am, some senile old fart like you? You know what he said?

Me: No idea.

Patient: He said, "You know, you're right! You're so sharp, you're a real cookie!" And I said, "I'm not a cookie, I'm a treat!" Doc, do you want a Bundt cake?

Me: I enjoy Bundt cakes for sure.

Patient: Well, since all those decrepits in my building never pick up the free coupon magazine, I take them. And the bakery across the way give out free mini Bundts with these coupons I found. I've been getting one a day for the past three weeks!

(*Patient gives me a coupon.*)

Me: Thanks! I'm glad these coupons aren't going to waste.

Patient: In fact, the other day, some old creepy guy tried to pick me up in the parking lot. Said he wanted to make sure I got to my car. That's a likely story. First of all, I'm much smarter than him, and second, he was at least seventy-five years old! I'm not interested in anyone over the age of fifty-five. Otherwise, they can't keep up.

Me: Wow. Well, you seem to have a lot of energy.

Patient: Well, doc, are we done here?

Me: I don't think we've started.

Seeing patients again . . .

Me: What brings you in here today?

Patient: I'm always off balance, always swaying side to side when I'm walking.

Me: How long has that been going on for?

Patient: The past couple of years or so.

Me: Anything that you can think of that may have set it off?

Patient: I started to drink more.

Me: Drink more what? Alcohol?

Patient: Yeah.

Me: Well, how much are you drinking?

Patient: Oh, not that much, four to five glasses.

Me: Sure. Glasses of what?

Patient: Vodka.

Me: Oh OK. How big is a glass?

Patient: Like a coffee mug. But I've been trying to cut back, but every time I do, I start to hear a sound in my ears.

Me: What type of sound? Like a buzzing or ringing?

Discontinue Leeches!!
And Other Stories from an ENT's Training

Patient: No, the symphony starts playing.

(*Long pause.*)

Me: The symphony starts playing? Like actual music?

Patient: Yeah, I don't know what it is, but it might be Bach. Possibly Beethoven.

Me: How long after you stop drinking does that start?

Patient: Like two days. But then I usually start drinking again, and it goes away.

Me: OK, so your problem isn't your ears, it's the alcohol. I think you're having early signs of DTs when you're trying to quit. And that's really, really dangerous, you could die. Who's your primary care doctor? If you really want this stuff to stop, you need to dry out.

Patient: No, I don't want to do that. As long as it's not my ears, I'm happy. Thanks! I'll see you later.

Have to send a package from work, so I go to find some packing tape

Me: Quick question . . . Do we have any packing tape around?

Secretary: Yeah, but it's kind of a process to get it.

Me: Really?

Secretary: Follow me.

(*Walk to the back room to a locked closet for which she has the key. Opens it and gets another key.*)

Me: Really?

Secretary: Just wait.

(*Walk to another locked office, which she opens with the key just obtained.*)

Me: Really?

(*Secretary starts to laugh. She reaches under the desk to a safe into which she puts a six-digit combination. She opens the safe and pulls out another key.*)

Me: What is happening right now?

Secretary: One more.

(*She opens a cabinet above the desk and pulls out the packing tape.*)

Secretary: Just make sure you bring it back afterward. It's a hot commodity.

Discontinue Leeches!!
And Other Stories from an ENT's Training

Me: Apparently! You know there're things like scalpels and needles that are a bit easier to get to than this packing tape, right?

Secretary: Well, we had a big issue with the packing tape a few years ago. I don't want to talk about it.

Me: Well, you have to tell me now!

Secretary: Another time. I should get back to work.

SEEING A LADY IN HER LATE FIFTIES FOR NASAL CONGESTION

Me: OK, I'm gonna take a look in your nose with a scope, so I'm going to give you a nasal spray to help numb and decongest things.

Lady: OK.

(*I spray her nose with the topical medication.*)

Lady, *after I'm done spraying*: Oh wow, what was that stuff?

Me: Oh, it's a mixture of lidocaine, a numbing medication, and phenylephrine, which is a decongestant. Sorry, it can taste kinda terrible.

Lady: No, no, it's not that. I feel great!

Me: Yeah, well, you have a lot of congestion because of your allergies, so this probably opened things up a bit for you.

Lady: I mean, it did that, but that reminds me of when I used to do cocaine! Feels exactly the same!

(*Long pause.*)

Me: You use cocaine? I didn't see that in your history.

Lady: Yeah, well, I used to party pretty hard in my day. Spent a fair amount of time at Studio 54 in the late '70s. They used to have it right next to the soap in the bathroom. You'd be dancing, and then go freshen up, do a line a coke, and be right back out there!

Me: Wow.

Discontinue Leeches!!
And Other Stories from an ENT's Training

Lady: My god, what am I doing telling you that? You're young enough to be my son! I don't do that stuff anymore. But oh man, that stuff you gave me just took me back!

(*Scope her and find she has run-of-the-mill allergies. Talk with her a bit about treatment and begin to wrap things up.*)

Lady, *winking*: You couldn't possibly just spray my nose one more time, could you?

Me: Nope, doesn't work that way. But you're welcome for letting you relive a bit of your youth.

FIELDING CALLS FROM PATIENTS OVER THE WEEKEND. PATIENT'S MOTHER CALLS ABOUT HER EIGHT YEAR-OLD KID WHO HAD A TONSILLECTOMY.

Mother: I gave him the liquid Motrin this morning, but he threw it up. He's still in pain, but he doesn't want to take of the liquid Motrin.

Me: OK, is he drinking fluid? Keeping things down?

Mother: Not for a couple of hours. He says his throat hurts too much.

Me: All right. Well, encourage him to drink as much as possible, and try the liquid Motrin again.

Mother: He really doesn't want to take it. Do you think I could give him a suppository?

(*Long pause.*)

Me: A suppository? I mean . . . you could. No offense, but you do know what a suppository is?

Mother: I do, but he really doesn't want to take anything by mouth, and he's complaining of pain.

Me: You could try, but I don't think an eight-year-old boy is necessarily going to go for a suppository. I'd still just encourage him to take stuff by mouth.

Mother: I'm going to try the suppository.

Discontinue Leeches!! And Other Stories from an ENT's Training

Me: OK. Do me a favor, tell him what a suppository is before you try to give it to him.

(*Ten minutes later get paged to call the mother back.*)

Mother: He started to cry when I told him about what the suppository was and agreed to take the liquid Motrin by mouth.

Me: Perfect. Sounds like you fixed him.

SEEING A CONSULT IN THE HOSPITAL. IN THE BED NEXT TO ME, A PASTOR IS TALKING WITH ANOTHER PATIENT.

Me, *to my patient*: So after scoping you, it looks like you have some nasal dryness and not airway obstruction like your admitting team thought.

My patient: Well, I could have told you that. Thanks for nothing!

Pastor, *to his patient*: It was so nice to talk with you. It can be tough giving up on medical treatment, but it's really about the quality of your life. And God will always help you through this until the time of your passing.

Pastor's patient: Thank you so much, it means a lot.

(*Pastor and I happen to walk out together. Pastor starts whistling Beethoven's Fifth Symphony.*)

Me: Sorry, I couldn't help but overhear. It sounded like you were talking to that patient about end-of-life care.

Pastor: Yeah, she and her family decided for hospice today.

Me: I imagine you get called a lot to those types of situations.

Pastor: Oh, all the time!

Me: How do you manage with that? I can imagine that it could be quite trying.

Pastor: I've been doing this for years, and it can be sometimes. But a lot of times they're just happy to be at peace with the world. And sometimes it's sharing a smile with them. And God always helps me through difficult times. I heard that patients can be kind of nasty to you. How do you deal with that?

Me: Well, I figure they're not happy to be in the hospital anyway, and I'm some sort of nameless face asking them to do something else. I'm fine if they want to take a bit of frustration out on me.

(*We walk in silence for a bit.*)

Me: Anyway, you're still whistling.

Pastor: You have to!

(*We get on an elevator together. Pastor looks at the carrying case for my flexible scope.*)

Pastor: What do you have in the case?

Me: Oh, that's my violin. See, when there's a code in the unit and it doesn't look like they're going to make it, they call me and I start playing Chopin's Funeral March.

(*Pastor and I share a look, and then he starts laughing loudly.*)

Pastor: Well, at least I know you have a sense of humor about what happens in this place.

Me: You have to!

SEEING PATIENTS AGAIN

Me: So what brings you in here today?

Patient: First, thank you for seeing me! I've read so much about you.

Me: No problem. What's going on?

Patient: I know you can help me.

Me: Well, I'll certainly try. What can I help you with?

Patient: I've been having headaches for about two months now.

Me: OK, anything happen two months ago that you can think of that set them off? Sinus issues? Allergies? Infections?

(*Long pause.*)

Patient: Oh no, nothing like that. I did electrocute myself though.

Me: What now? How did you do that?

Patient: Oh, the usual way.

Me: There's a usual way to electrocute yourself?

Patient: My toaster wasn't working. I checked all the connections in the toaster. Then I looked at the plug. I tried unplugging it, but it was stuck. So I tried to use a knife to get the prongs out of the socket, and I got a huge shock. Ever since then, I've been having bad headaches and weird things with my vision, and my left arm has been tingling.

Me: Um . . . did you go to the hospital?

Patient: I felt really bad that day, but I looked it up on the Internet, and it said I'd be fine.

Me: But you're having headaches and vision changes.

Patient: I know, but I called four or five other doctors, and they all told me I'd be fine.

Me: Four or five other doctors told you that you'd be fine after you electrocuted yourself?

Patient: Well . . . no. They told me to get checked out.

Me: Did you see any of them?

Patient: No, I decided to see you instead.

Me: OK, great! I'll take a look at you, but I really think you need to see a neurologist.

Patient: But you deal with the head, right? And my head is aching. Like a headache!

Me: Sure, yeah, certain parts. I'll make sure there's nothing going on with your ears, nose, or throat. After that, probably a neurologist to make sure you don't have brain damage.

Patient: Electrocuting yourself can cause brain damage?

Me: Yeah.

Patient: So the Internet lied to me.

Me: I really wouldn't trust your health to the Internet.

Patient: Are you lying to me?

Me: Absolutely not.

SEEING A TWENTY-SOMETHING FEMALE PATIENT FOR NASAL OBSTRUCTION. SCOPE HER TO FIND A LARGE POLYP EXTENDING FROM THE MAXILLARY SINUS THROUGH THE BACK OF THE NOSE.

Me, *going over the video of the scope*: You have what's called an antrochoanal polyp. That's just the medical term for a large polyp going from the maxillary sinus—that's the sinus in your cheek—to the back of the nose. It's filling up everything back there, so that's why you have difficulty breathing.

Patient: That's my anus? Wait, I have anal polyps? You can see that far?

(*Long pause as I stare at the patient.*)

Me: Well, that would be something if I could see anal polyps looking through your nose. It's antrochoanal. *Antro* for the opening of the maxillary sinus, and *choana*, fancy term for the entrance to the back of the nose. Nowhere near the anus. Can't really see the anus or rectum or colon through the nose.

Patient, *turns beet red*: OMG, I'm so embarrassed. That's so gross though!

Me: It is kinda gross. But it's OK. We can do a surgery through your nose to remove the polyp and any of the diseased mucosal lining.

Patient, *looking relieved*: Oh, I'm so glad! So I don't have anal polyps?

Me: Not that I can tell, but you'll have to see another type of doctor for those sorts of issues.

Waiting in Checkout Line at the Grocery Store

Lady in front of me: Excuse me, Dr. Patel?

Me: Um . . . yes?

Lady: Oh wow, this is like fate that I ran into you! You saw me a few months ago about a stuffed nose.

(*I have no recollection of who this person is.*)

Me: Oh OK, I hope you're feeling better.

Lady: I really am.

Me: Great, I'm glad I could help you.

(*Lady looks at my groceries.*)

Lady: I see you're buying some salt. Don't doctors always say salt is bad for you? So why are you buying it?

Me, *clearly uncomfortable*: Because I like salt on my food.

Lady: Oh OK. Listen, I'm so happy I ran into you. I've been having this thing going on with my ears. Could you take a look at them?

(*Lady begins to turn her head toward me for me to look at her left ear.*)

Me: I'm sorry, I'm going to stop you right there. I don't necessarily think the checkout line is the best place to be examining your ears. I'm happy to see you in the office whenever you'd like.

Lady: Oh sure, definitely! Maybe you can stick that scope in my nose again. I'll call tomorrow!

(*Lady finishes checking out and leaves. Cashier has been listening to the entire conversation.*)

Cashier: Does that happen to you often?

Me: Not very often. But . . . it's enough for me to never want to come here again.

Difference between residency and attending life

(Seeing a dizzy patient as the last patient of the day as a resident)

Me, *picking up chart, to myself or sometimes to another resident*: FUCK, ANOTHER FUCKING DIZZY PATIENT.* I cannot fucking stand dizzy patients. I'm goddamn exhausted, I want to go home, but I have to see this patient and then wait for the attending. It's going take for-fucking-ever. The patient's going to start yelling at me. I NEED TO SHOTGUN SOME SKITTLES AND A DIET DR. PEPPER!**

(*Essentially end up seeing the patient, rushing through a history and physical, waiting another hour for the attending, I'm unhappy, the patient's unhappy, the attending's unhappy, and everyone leaves angry.*)

*If it is not obvious, I used to swear like a drill sergeant.

**This was my diet on most Wednesday afternoons for four years.

(Seeing a dizzy patient as the last patient of the day as an attending)

Me, *to no one in particular*: Ugh, another dizzy patient. I'm tired and I want to go home, but whatever.

(*See patient, takes about thirty minutes, and send her out. I walk over the office manager.*)

Me: Can you change my schedule so I don't see any dizzy patients during my last hour in the office?

Office manager: Why not?

Me: I don't like seeing dizzy patients. It's not my cup of tea. But I'll see them if I have to. But I don't want to see them at the end of the day. I don't have the mental wherewithal late in the afternoon to deal with it. It's essentially a patient care issue. I'm not giving the best care to dizzy patients if they're the last patients of the day. Does that make sense?

Office manager: Definitely. We'll block your schedule accordingly.

Me: That was surprisingly easy.

Office manager: Well, we like to keep our docs happy.

Seeing patients yet again, this time a sixty-six-year-old lady for hearing loss

Me: So it looks like you have some amount of hearing loss in the high frequencies. Nothing that I wouldn't expect for noise exposure over the course of your lifetime and age-related hearing loss.

Patient: Let me tell you, it sucks getting old.

Me: Happens to all of us unfortunately.

Patient: Things seem to just fall apart. Your body hurts, you forget things, you have to take all these pills—it's terrible! It's like that line from that old Beatles song, you know, "What a drag it is getting old."

(*Slight pause.*)

Me: That's a Rolling Stones song. "Mother's Little Helper."

Patient: Wait, are you sure?

Me: Yeah, "She goes running for the shelter of a mother's little helper . . ."

Patient: Yeah, that's the one.

Me: Definitely a Rolling Stones song, not the Beatles. Seems like you've just demonstrated one of those memory issues.

Patient: Oh, this is the worst! I'm getting schooled on rock and roll by someone who's younger than my daughter!

Me: It is what it is. Anything else I can help you with today?

Patient: No, you've done enough.

Seeing older patient for removal of an epistat, a giant nasal packing for nosebleeds

Me: Hello, sir, I'm here to remove the packing.

Patient: Oh, thank God! Is it going to hurt?

Me: Well, it won't be comfortable. But a lot better than going in.

Patient: You're telling me! I wanted to punch that other doctor who put it in.

Me: Yeah, that's how it works though. Sometimes I have to be the bad cop and shove those things into noses, and sometimes I get to the good cop and take them out. Today I get to be the good cop.

(*Take packing out.*)

Patient: I feel so much better. Say, you look to be a young feller. That makes me so happy to see young folk becoming doctors. We need more of you.

Me: Well, I'm glad I could help you out. Hopefully this won't happen again.

Patient: Well, I'm tickled pink to have met you, sonny!

(*Turns beet red.*)

Patient: I'm sorry you remind me of my grandson. I meant to say "sir."

(*Considers it again.*)

Patient: Actually, I mean to say, thank you, doctor!

Me: You're very welcome, and don't worry about it. We'll see you later.

(Sometimes it's worth it.)

SEEING A TWENTY-THREE-YEAR-OLD PATIENT FOR CERUMEN IMPACTION

Patient: I was told by my doctor I have a lot of earwax. He told me to come here to get it taken out. He tried to flush out the ear, but it didn't work. I never want to have that done again.

Me: OK, let's take a look.

(*Wax in both ear canals.*)

Me: OK, since you didn't like the irrigation, I can use a vacuum and a little scoop to take this stuff out. It looks pretty soft, so it should come out pretty easily.

Patient, *looks apprehensive*: Is it going to hurt?

Me: It shouldn't, but it can be a bit uncomfortable. If it hurts, we can stop.

(*I get the suction and curette ready and turn around to see the patient with a death grip on the chair and a scrunched-up pained expression on his face, which is turning beet red.*)

Me: Um, what are you doing?

Patient: I'm getting ready.

Me: OK . . .

(*Patient starts saying Hail Marys. I reach down and pull back gently on his ear to look in with the otoscope. Patient screams as if I've gored him with a harpoon.*)

Me: What's wrong?

Discontinue Leeches!! And Other Stories from an ENT's Training

Patient: That hurt so much! Did you get the wax out?

Me: I haven't even looked in your ear yet, much less taken anything out. I don't understand, you let me look in your ears not more than twenty seconds ago.

Patient: Oh OK. (*Starts saying Our Fathers.*)

(*I look in his ear and then raise the suction. Patient screams again and then gets up out of the chair and starts pacing around.*)

Patient, *yelling*: That hurt so much! Did you get it out?

Me: I still haven't done anything.

Patient: Well, I can't take this pain. I'm leaving!

(*Patient walks out. Medical assistant walks in.*)

MA: What did you do to that guy?

Me: Not a thing!

IN BETWEEN SEEING PATIENTS

Medical assistant: So I heard being a resident is hard.

Me: Yes, it is.

MA: What's it like?

Me: What's it like? I can try to tell you what the mind-set of a resident is . . .

(*Chief year. Six hours into a free flap case, and we've just finished the resection. Attending is feeling somewhat generous.*)

Attending: Amit, you did a not-terrible job on that neck dissection. Go get something to drink really quickly, but hurry back, we need to start on the flap.

(*I scrub out and run downstairs to the cafeteria. I get something to drink, but all of a sudden, the cafeteria is filled with police. After a few minutes, I walk up to one of them.*)

Me: Um, what's going on?

Policeman: A prisoner escaped from one of the floors. We're locking down the hospital to look for him. So you can't leave from here because we're concerned he might attack someone.

Me: Fuck.

(*Medical assistant interrupts.*)

MA: So you had to stay down there?

Me: Well, I had two options. Stay down there for an indeterminate amount of time, knowing that my attending was going to yell at me more and more the longer he had to wait, or wait until the cops weren't looking and risk getting taken hostage or murdered to get back to the operating room as soon as possible.

MA: So what did you do?

Me: I waited until the cops weren't looking, and then I ran back to the operating room.

MA: So what happened?

Me: Well, obviously, I didn't get murdered, but my attending wasn't happy about me being so late back to the case. He revoked my food privileges for the rest of the rotation. But that's what goes through a resident's mind. Literally risk getting murdered because you're more afraid of your attending yelling at you or being disappointed in you.

MA: That sounds awful!

Me: It was. And is.

> ithcy ear and has been having pooping ear, h

I blame falling educational standards and lack of public school funding for this patient complaint. Nobody really places importance on basics such as spelling anymore. While a lot of shit does come out of the ear (please see previous rants on earwax), poop does not. And although I would have loved to diagnose the world's first colocochlear fistula, the reality was much more mundane.

Seeing a nice older Indian lady (approximately seventy-five years old) for hearing loss

Patient: Oh, you're such a nice young doctor.

Me: Thank you. I'm glad I could help you today.

Patient: Let me ask you something. You know, my father had hearing loss.

Me: Oh, really?

Patient: Yes, yes, when he was very young, he lost hearing in his left ear. He went to all the specialists all over India, and no one could tell him what was wrong.

Me: OK.

Patient: Then he went to Juhu beach, you know, in Mumbai.

Me: OK.

Patient: And he went to one of those *kaan saaf wallahs* (professional ear cleaners) on the street. And he pulled a looong stringy thing out of the ear. Then he could hear!

Me: OK.

Patient, *looking at me expectantly*: So what was that?

Me: I have no idea, but it sounds like wax.

Patient: But he said it wasn't wax. It was a long stringy thing.

Me: OK, but I still have no idea. Plus this was ninety years ago. And in India.

Patient: Oh well, I thought you might know.

Me: Sorry to disappoint.

(Sometimes I don't have all the answers.)

Seeing a patient for "ear issues"

Me: So what brings you in here today?

Patient: My ears have been bothering me.

Me: OK, how so? Like you can't hear out of them? Drainage? Infections? Pain?

Patient: Well, it's going to sound a bit weird.

Me, *leaning forward in anticipation*: Oh OK, what's going on?

Patient: My ears itch every now and then.

(*Long pause.*)

Me: That's it? They itch?

Patient: Yeah, isn't that so bizarre though?

Me: Ummmm, not really.

(*Turn to my computer and type a bit of the history and then turn back to the patient.*)

Me: I mean, if you told me that you thought you had a hamster in your ear or you thought there was a little orchestra playing in there, THAT would be weird. Itchy ears are fine. You're allowed to have itchy ears, very common complaint.

Patient, *laughs*: Oh OK, good. Wait, have other people told you stuff like that before?

Me: Oh definitely. So your ear itchiness, very run-of-the-mill.

IN THE HOSPITAL FOR A TONGUE-TIE CONSULT

Me, *to nursing staff*: Hello, my name's Dr. Patel. Someone here called about this tongue-tie release earlier today.

Nurse: Wow, you came? Didn't expect to see you tonight.

Me: Why wouldn't I come?

Nurse: Well, some do and some don't.

Me: Eh, I enjoy doing these things. Plus I get to poke the babies in their bellies. Always fun.

(*We go to see the patient. I get consent from the mom, and we wheel the bassinet out of the room.*)

Nurse: Gosh, this baby is cute. Look at those cheeks!

Me: He's a cute baby for sure. But then again, they all are, aren't they?

Nurse, *looking around, presumably for parents*: Nope, there are some real uggos. Obviously, we don't tell the parents that. But we have our favorites.

Me: I've always suspected. Don't worry, your secret is safe with me.

(We get to the procedure room, and I set up for the tongue-tie release.)

Nurse: Can I ask you something?

Me: Sure.

Discontinue Leeches!!
And Other Stories from an ENT's Training

Nurse: This baby had a circumcision done by the OB. That seems like a much more complicated and risky procedure than this tongue-tie release, which seems to take you five seconds.

Me: OK. What's the question?

Nurse: Well, why can't the OB just do the tongue-tie release?

Me, *in a whisper*: Shhh, be quiet! You'll ruin it all for the ENTs! We get an easy five bucks for this procedure. We know the OBs COULD do it, but then we'd never get to come by and poke these babies in their bellies. And then what would we do?

Nurse: Oh OK. And don't worry, your secret is safe with me.

Me: Perfect.

(Nearly) every teenager/early twenties tonsillectomy patient after discussing risks of the procedure

Me: So the number-one thing patients complain about after tonsillectomy is pain. It's definitely worse the older you are. I can't stress this enough, but it will be the WORST sore throat you've ever had. Pain medications will help, and I'll prescribe a strong one, but you are going to be completely miserable afterward.

Patient: Yeah, I've heard that. I also read about it on the Internet.

Me: Definitely. So again, it is going to be painful. You're not going to want to go out, see friends, play sports, eat hamburgers, anything. As long as you're drinking enough fluids, that's all that matters.

Patient: Yeah, I got it.

(*A few weeks later, seeing patient in the office preop.*)

Me: Just to remind you again, it's really, really going to be painful. No overstatement.

Patient: Yeah, you'd mentioned that last time.

Me: I just want to make sure you understand.

(*Next week, see the patient in holding right before the operation.*)

Me: Any other questions or concerns? I know we've gone over the risks and benefits quite a bit, and again, it's going to be very painful after the operation. Most pain is within the first few days, but again, like we talked about, you're going to be pretty miserable for a week, maybe two.

Patient: Yes, you've told me.

Me: OK, just making sure.

(*At some point postop day 1–3, phone call from patient.*)

Patient: My throat hurts so much!

Me: Yeah, but we talked about this! You knew it was going to hurt. A lot.

Patient: Well, I didn't think it would be THIS bad.

Me: (*Le SIGH.*)

SEEING AN INDIAN GUY FOR NOSEBLEEDS

Patient, *thick accent*: Well, buddy, I really need to know why this is happening.

Me: Well, we'll try to figure it out. Any trauma to the nose?

Patient: Well, you know, right, *bhai*?

(*Bhai* is Gujarati for "brother.")

Me: No, I don't. Did you hit your nose? Break it?

Patient, *leans in and whispers*: You know how all Indian people pick their noses, right?

Me, *leaning in*: No, they don't. But it sounds like you do.

Patient: Oh, come now, bhai, you pick your nose, right, boss?

Me: I really don't pick my nose.

Patient: Well, you know, Indian people pick their noses. Like this!

(*Patient sticks his finger in his nose and then flicks it forward toward me, flinging mucus directly at me, which fortunately misses. Nose starts to bleed.*)

Patient: You see, it always starts when I do that.

Me: Well, I figured out why your nose is bleeding.

Seeing an Older Patient for Hearing Loss

Me: How long have you been having hearing loss for?

Patient, *yelling*: LONG TIME! I'M HERE FOR THE HEARING TEST!

Me: OK, we'll get to that. I need to make sure there's nothing else going on with the ears in terms of infections, earwax, or anything else.

Patient, *looks at me strangely*: WHAT DO YOU THINK OF TRUMP?

(*Long pause while I consider my response to keep things as apolitical as possible.*)

Me: I didn't vote for him. So . . .

Patient, *gives me a disgusted look*: SO YOU VOTED FOR HILLARY?

Me: Yes, I did. Can I just examine your ears?

(*Ears are normal. He goes and gets his hearing test and gets put back in a room. I walk in a few minutes later.*)

Patient, *thinking he's speaking under his breath but is actually talking in a normal voice*: Huh, now here comes this Arab immigrant to tell me what's what. This country's gone to shit.

(*I give him a look.*)

Patient: OH, CAN YOU HEAR ME?

Me: Yes, I can. First off, I'm not Arab. My family's from India originally. Second, I'm an American citizen born in this country. Third, it's pretty common with hearing loss to talk louder than you think you are talking. Your hearing test shows you have a moderate to severe loss on both sides. You're here for hearing loss. I think you should get hearing aids. Maybe then you can try to keep your views to yourself.

Patient: CAN I GO NOW?

Me: Yes, you can go.

(*Patient leaves. Medical assistant comes in.*)

MA: So is he coming here to get his hearing aids?

Me: He can, but I hope not. Never want to see him again.

SEEING A NINETY-FIVE-YEAR-OLD LADY FOR HEARING LOSS, BROUGHT IN BY HER GRANDDAUGHTER

Me: So I understand you've had hearing loss for a long time.

Patient: You got it! I've been using these aids for twenty years, and they broke. But I don't need 'em!

Granddaughter: Gran, you do need them. You never hear us.

Patient: Well, maybe it's because I don't like what you're saying!

Granddaughter: Maybe.

Me: We won't get into issues like that. Let me take a look at you.

(*Put on a pair of gloves.*)

Patient: Oh my! Those are some nice gloves! I need gloves like that. See my hands? They're delicate! They get all cracked and dry when I do my gardening.

(*I look in her ears and take out some wax. Everything is normal, and I go over the hearing test, which shows a moderate to severe loss on both sides.*)

Me: OK, this test suggests that you might do well with hearing aids. If the other ones are broken, you should look into getting new aids. The technology is always changing. But it's a decision that you have to make.

Patient: I don't know. What's worth listening to these days? The news? There's that crazy man they elected, and all he has to say is nonsense! I just turn it off. I don't need to hear that!

(*Patient looks down at my gloved hands again.*)

Patient: Gosh, those are some nice-looking gloves.

Granddaughter: Will you stop asking him about his gloves?

Me: I'll make a deal with you. I'll give you this box of gloves for your gardening if you consider getting new hearing aids.

Patient: Wow, one-stop shopping! That's great. You're such a nice young doctor.

Me: I try.

Patient: I'll look into the hearing aids. As long as I don't have to listen to that crazy man.

Me: Only if you don't want to.

Patient, *as she's leaving*: You know, we just had a very good president.

Me: Oh, I know.

(*Medical assistant comes in.*)

MA: Dr. Patel, what happened to all your gloves?

Me: I gave them to that lady who just left.

MA: What? Why?

Me: Part of a deal. Also, she's lived to ninety-five and is probably entitled to some freebies.

SEEING A TEENAGE GIRL FOR EAR FULLNESS, WHICH TURNS OUT TO BE WAX

Patient: I can't believe this is happening to me. Just the thought of it sitting in there grosses me out. I'm so clean otherwise!

Me: It's OK, nothing to worry about. I'll remove it.

Patient: OMG, like an operation? I can't handle that.

Me: Not like an operation, but I'll use a little vacuum to suck the wax out of your ear.

Patient, *apprehensive*: I'm not going to like this.

Me: Don't worry, you're gonna do great!

(*I use a suction to clear a pretty decent plug of wax out of her left ear, which I grab off the tip of the suction with a four-by-four gauze. Patient cringed throughout the entire procedure and is slightly flushed and sweaty.*)

Patient, *eyes closed*: Is it over?

Me: Yup.

Patient, *opens eyes*: What was in there? Can I see it?

(*I hand her the piece of gauze with the wax.*)

Patient: OMG, that's the grossest thing ever! That was in me?

Me: Yup.

Patient: I feel a little faint. Can I sit here for a little bit and close my eyes?

Me: Sure, I have to finish my note up anyway.

(*I turn away and finish up my note. I turn back to find the patient with a huge brown streak across her forehead.*)

Me: Um, did you just wipe that wax across your forehead?

Patient, *eyes widen*: Oh no, I was sweaty, and I completely forgot that was in that tissue you handed me!

(*Patient starts retching.*)

Me: OK, well, here's a tissue to wipe that stuff off your head, and here's a basin in case you throw up. I'm gonna go check on another patient, and I'll be back to see you in a couple of minutes.

Patient: I'm such an idiot!

Me: That was embarrassing for you.

Patient: I know!

(Never going to let another patient see their wax again.)

SEEING A YOUNGISH GUY FOR POSSIBLE HEARING LOSS

Me: Have you noticed you've had hearing loss at all?

Patient: I don't think so. But you know, people always are telling me I'm talking loud, so you get to wondering, you know, am I deaf?

Me: I understand. Who's telling you you're having problems hearing?

Patient: My wife mostly. She says I'm yelling all the time, but who knows? We just moved into a bigger house, and sometimes I have to yell across from another room. Plus, I'm just a loud person. It runs in my family, you know, my father is loud, my uncles are loud. I'm Spanish, you know? We're a loud people!

Me: Fair enough.

(*Clean out some wax from the ears and send him for his hearing test, which is normal.*)

Patient: How did I do?

Me: You have perfect hearing on both sides.

Patient: Man, I knew it! Can I get a copy of that? So that my wife stops nagging me?

Me: Definitely, but I'm afraid that might open up a whole other can of worms for you.

(*Patient considers it for a moment.*)

Patient: You know, you're right. But at least I have good hearing!

Me: Absolutely. See you later.

Attempting to schedule a septoplasty (fixing the midportion of the nose) for a patient

Surgical coordinator: Did you get a CT scan on this patient?

Me: No, I didn't think it was necessary. He has no sinus issues, no recurrent infections, and pretty obvious deviation to the right along with some turbinate hypertrophy when I scoped him. And he has problems breathing through that right side and has tried all sorts of nasal sprays and everything. He's pretty miserable about it, that's why I think the surgery would help him.

Surgical coordinator: His insurance company is denying the surgery because there was no CT scan done.

Me: Really?

Surgical coordinator: Yeah, some insurance companies absolutely require a CT scan before you do a septoplasty.

Me: Can I talk to them?

(*She gets me on the phone with the insurance company, and I explain the situation.*)

Insurance: Yeah, we won't approve the surgery without the CT scan.

Me: OK, I think it's unnecessary radiation, but I don't want the guy to pay out of pocket for the surgery either. He can't afford that. I'll order the CT scan.

(*I order the CT scan, and a couple of days later, my medical assistant comes to see me.*)

MA: Remember that guy you ordered the CT scan for? The insurance company denied it.

Discontinue Leeches!!
And Other Stories from an ENT's Training

Me: What? They're the ones that wanted me to order it in the first place.

(Call up the insurance company again for a peer-to-peer review.)

Doctor: So why exactly did you order this CT scan? You're not documenting any symptoms consistent with allergies or chronic sinusitis, only a deviated septum and turbinate hypertrophy.

Me: I know. I didn't want the CT scan in the first place, only to correct his deviated septum and reduce the size of the turbinates. I don't think he has underlying sinus disease based on my history or physical. But your insurance company denied the surgery because I had no CT scan. Now you're telling me you won't approve a CT scan.

Doctor: Oh man, another one of these.

Me: So this has happened before to you? Sounds like a catch-22 situation to me.

Doctor: Yeah, it's happened before.

Me: OK, I think it's something you should figure out. Because now I have to explain to this guy why I can't schedule his surgery, and he's gonna think I'm crazy. And I'm gonna refer him to your company. And you can explain to him why.

SEEING A TWENTY-SOMETHING-YEAR-OLD BLONDE FOR CHRONIC TONSILLITIS, WHO CAME IN WITH HER BOYFRIEND

Me: How many times has this happened to you over the course of the past year?

Patient: A lot!

Me: OK, a lot. Give or take, try to put a number on it.

Patient: Probably about twenty or so.

Me: Wow, twenty times?

Boyfriend: It hasn't been twenty times. (*To me*) Don't listen to her, she's a blonde. You know how it is.

(*I give the boyfriend a weird look.*)

Patient: Well, it's been different things. Sometimes it's just a cough and cold without a sore throat. Sometimes it's allergies and runny nose. Sometimes it's a bad sore throat.

Me: OK, how many sore throats have you had?

Patient: Probably like six or seven then. And they keep swabbing it, and it's strep throat every time!

Boyfriend: See, you have to tell him things like that. (*To me*) Goes along with the blonde thing.

(*Again, give the boyfriend a weird look.*)

Discontinue Leeches!!
And Other Stories from an ENT's Training

Patient, *to boyfriend*: Stop saying that!

(*I finish up the history and physical, which is consistent with recurrent acute tonsillitis, and am discussing tonsillectomy. The boyfriend keeps interjecting about her being blonde.*)

Me: So it's very painful afterward, essentially the worst sore throat you've ever had, and we'll keep you on some strong pain medication. But you will be quite miserable.

Patient: I have a pretty high tolerance for pain. Plus I just want these infections to go away!

Me: OK, so maybe you'll be better than most with this, but I'm just telling you what to expect.

Boyfriend, *to patient*: You really have no idea.

Me, *turn to boyfriend, with a smile*: Oh, have you had your tonsils out?

Boyfriend: No. But I've heard things.

Me: So you don't really have any idea of what you're talking about because you have no frame of reference. (*To patient, again with a smile*) You know, all that stuff about being blonde is utter nonsense. It's like saying someone is less intelligent because they wear red shoes or, say, because of skin color. It's ridiculous.

Patient, *laughing*: Oh, I know. I get better grades in classes than him anyway, so he's just jealous.

Boyfriend: Hey!

Me, *to boyfriend*: Wow, is that true about the grades?

Boyfriend: I'm not saying.

Me: All right, I think we've settled things. Let's get you scheduled for that tonsillectomy!

Walk into a lunch sponsored by a drug rep who is promoting an inhaled steroid

Me, *to drug rep*: Hi, my name's Amit Patel. I'm one of the ENTs here in the practice. Thanks for bringing food. What are you talking about today?

Drug rep, *eyes get really wide*: I'm not allowed to talk to you.

Me: What, me specifically?

Drug rep: I'm only allowed to talk to the allergist on staff.

Me: What, why?

Drug rep, *holding both hands out in stop gesture*: Listen, I know you guys like to use the inhaled steroids off label for whatever you do, but I can't legally or ethically talk about that stuff.

Me: Um. OK. I wasn't going to ask you to do anything ethically ambiguous.

Drug rep: It's best not even to get into the conversation.

Me: Awesome, I can still have this pizza, though, right?

Drug rep: Yes.

(*Get some pizza and go to the table and sit down.*)

Drug rep: I didn't mean to be rude before, but I just don't want to get into trouble, you know, ethically.

Me: Whatever, it's fine. No big deal.

Drug rep: We can talk about anything else though.

Me: Sure, OK. Like what?

Drug rep: I don't know. I'm only prepared to talk about this drug.

Me: Great.

(*Eat the rest of lunch in silence.*)

Seeing a Fifteen-Year-Old Wrestler Brought in by His Mother for Auricular Hematoma (Blood Collection in the External Ear)

Me: So when did this happen?

Patient: About six weeks ago.

Me: You've had a fluid collection there for six weeks? Did you get it drained?

Patient: No, I was in the middle of the season, and I didn't want to interrupt it.

(*I look over at the mother.*)

Mom: I tried, but he refused. Said it didn't bother him. But we're here now.

Me: Any fevers, chills? Anything drain out of it?

Patient: Nope.

Me: Does your ear look normal to you?

Patient: It's a bit lumpy.

(*Examine the patient. The area where the hematoma was is now fibrotic and scarred down, essentially a cauliflower ear. But it doesn't look terrible.*)

Me: Well, there's no fluid collection there now, but it is a bit scarred down, which has affected the appearance of the ear slightly. Honestly, you should have gotten this drained when it first happened to prevent this from occurring. Plus sometimes the fluid collection can get infected, and then it can turn into a real mess. And you have to wear headgear when wrestling to try to protect the ear.

Mom: So there's nothing to drain? We came in too late?

Me: Nothing to drain, and a little late to come in for this. I can send you along to a plastic surgeon to look into resculpting the ear if you'd like.

Mom: So he's DEFORMED?

Patient: Mom, relax, it's fine. You're always complaining how long my hair is, but now I have a reason to have it long. It'll cover up my ear a bit.

Me: I wouldn't say deformed, that's a pretty strong word. It's not the worst-looking ear, but you can tell if you look at it closely that there's some scarring and irregularity to it. Again, I can send you to a plastic surgeon if you want.

Patient: Nah, I don't care about how my ear looks.

Mom: YOU HAVE TO LISTEN TO THE DOCTOR! YOU DID THIS TO YOURSELF! YOU HAVE TO CARE!

Patient: Mom, stop! It's fine.

Mom: I DON'T WANT YOU TO HAVE LONG HAIR! YOU MIGHT NOT CARE ABOUT YOUR EAR, BUT I CARE! I'M YOUR MOTHER!

Me: OK, well, if there's nothing else, you guys are good to go. But if it happens again, please call and see me right away to drain it and prevent more scarring or further changes in the ear.

Patient: Nah, it's cool, I'll just pop it myself.

Mom: ARE YOU CRAZY! YOU'RE NOT DOING THAT! YOU'RE COMING BACK HERE!

Me: All right, fair enough. Have a good day!

Seeing an older patient for postnasal drip. Walk into the room, and before I can introduce myself, the patient pipes up.

Patient, *stares at me for a second*: Wait, are you the doctor?

Me: Hello, yes, I'm Dr. Patel.

Patient: Hello. (*Thinks for a second and then clasps his hands in front of him*) Or should I say, *namaste*?

Me, *rolling eyes JUST slightly*: Yeah, you could say that too. Or *bienvenidos* for that matter. Out of curiosity, what would you have done if I weren't the doctor?

Patient: Probably the same thing.

Me: OK, so what brings you in here today?

Patient: I'm always dripping from my nose. All the time. I've had CT scans, allergy tests, everything, and everything always comes back normal! The only thing that's wrong with me is I got a case of pneumonia last week that I'm taking these steroids and antibiotics for from my pulmonologist.

Me: OK, but your nasal drip started before the pneumonia? It's an ongoing issue?

Patient: For years now!

(*Nothing else on history, examine the patient; nothing seems to be going on, so I diagnose vasomotor rhinitis.*)

Discontinue Leeches!!
And Other Stories from an ENT's Training

Me: It doesn't seem to be an infection or allergies or really related to any irritants. There is a condition called vasomotor rhinitis where you can have a constant clear drip of mucus from the nose, which sounds very much like what's going on in you.

Patient: Would it help if you saw what antibiotics I'm taking?

Me: Um, sure, I'll take a look.

(*Patient hands me three bottles, two with pills and one with a clear viscous liquid.*)

Me, *going through them*: OK, these pills are Levaquin. These are prednisone, and this one says Tessalon Perles, but it's filled with liquid.

Patient: Oh, right, that's my mucus sample from this morning. I thought you might want to have it.

Me, *putting it down quickly*: Nope. That's all right.

Patient: Hm, maybe I should give that to my lung doctor?

Me: Sure, you can have it back. I don't want it.

Patient: Actually, you keep it. I can always make more.

(*Patient winks at me.*)

Me: That's gross.

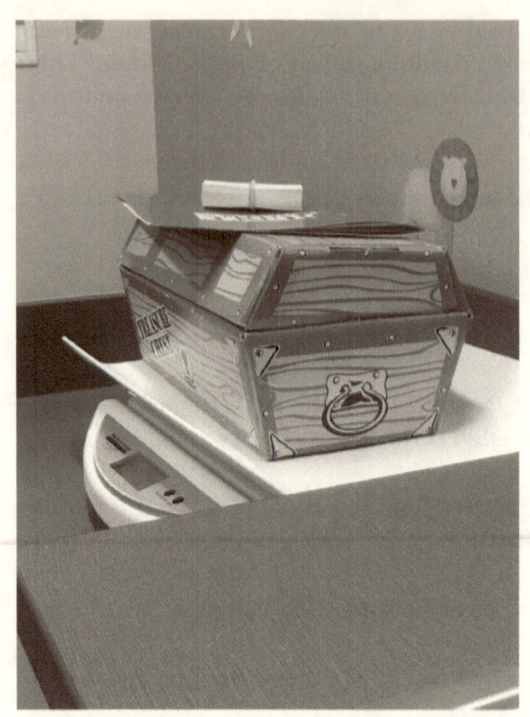

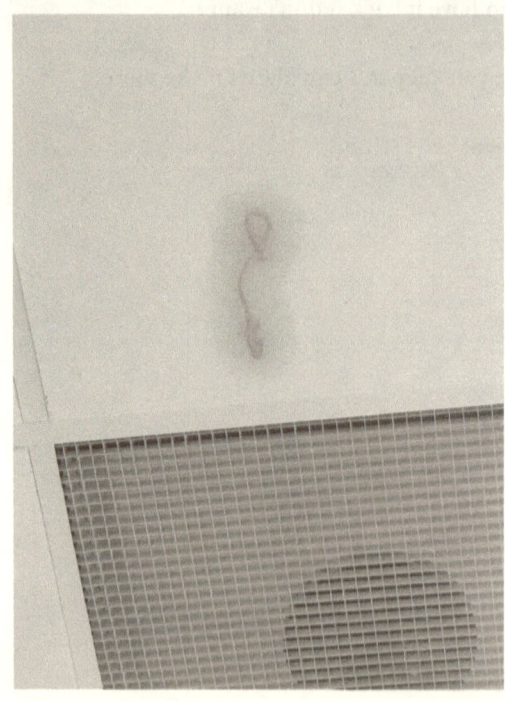

EVERY NOW AND AGAIN I GO OUT TO PROMOTE THE PRACTICE TO FAMILY PRACTICE PHYSICIANS, INTERNISTS, PEDIATRICIANS, AND URGENT CARE CENTERS, AND SO ON AND SO FORTH. TODAY I VISITED A NEW PEDIATRICIAN IN TOWN, AND SHE PUTS ME IN A ROOM WITH THIS BOX (SEE PICTURE 1).

Me: Oh wow, a treasure chest!

Pediatrician: Yeah, it's filled with all sorts of toys. Want to have a look?

Me: Oh definitely.

(*Look through the box and find all sorts of toy dinosaurs, little dolls, puzzles, etc.*)

Pediatrician: You know, you're welcome to take one if you want.

Me: I mean, I wouldn't say no to one of those toy dinosaurs because dinosaurs are awesome, but I should really leave them for the kids.

Pediatrician: All right. You know, it's tough knowing what to put into these boxes.

Me: What do you mean?

Pediatrician: Look up.

(*Look up [see picture 2].*)

Me: That's one of those sticky throw toys, isn't it?

Pediatrician: Yup. I thought they were a good idea, but then as soon as some kids got them, up they went.

Me: Not great.

Pediatrician: Yeah, we also used to have these little slingshot things in there too, but those were a disaster as well.

Me: I can imagine. That looks like it's been up there awhile. You going to take it down?

Pediatrician: Nope, going to leave it up there as a reminder.

Me: Awesome.

Ear foreign body part 1— call from the ER

ED doc: Hey, so we have this kid here. She has a bead stuck in her left ear.

Me: OK.

ED doc: Mom took her to a couple of ERs yesterday, and they couldn't get it out. So she went home and called the pediatrician, who told her to call an ENT. The ENT told them to come to this emergency room.

Me: Wow, the ENT referred them to an ER that they don't cover? Awesome.

ED doc: Yeah, well, we tried a few times, but it's really lodged in there.

Me: Can you guys do conscious sedation?

ED doc: No, we're not set up for that.

Me: OK, I'll come take a look.

(*Go into hospital and see the kid, who's obviously frightened as to what's happening. More about the history tomorrow, but I look in her left ear and see a white bead.*)

Me, *to kid*: So do you think you'll let me try again to get this bead out of your ear?

(*Kid bursts into tears and buries her head into mom's shoulder.*)

Me: OK! (*To mom*) We'll take her to the operating room. It'll be reasonably quick. Just give her some gas via a mask and pull this thing out. There's no sense in trying this down here. She's been through enough.

(*Go out to ED desk.*)

ED doc: Wow! That was quick. You got it out?

Me: No way, going to the OR.

ED doc: You can't do it here? We can hold her down if you'd like. I can get a couple of people to help out.

Me: What? I really don't enjoy torturing kids. I think it'll be easier on everyone involved if I just take her to the OR.

ED doc, *slightly disappointed*: Hm, I guess you're right.

Ear foreign body part 2—the history

Seeing a kid who has a bead stuck in her ear. Kid is there with her mother, who has an obvious accent, and her grandmother, who has one of those faces that looks like it can go from kind to scary very quickly. As an aside, I think all grandmothers can do this.

Me, *asking kid*: How did that bead get in there? Did you put it in there?

(*Kid shakes her head.*)

Mom: We took her to get her hair done last week, and they put those hair beads in her hair. After we found this thing in her ear, we looked in her bed and saw a couple of those beads by her pillow. So maybe one of them broke off and got stuck in her ear.

(*Look at the kid. She has no beads in her hair, and the hair is uneven.*)

Me, *pointing at hair*: Out of curiosity, did they only put a few beads in the hair? I don't see any right now.

(*Grandmother speaks up for the first time in a foreign language. Mom and grandmother talk rapidly back and forth for a few seconds, while grandmother makes a scissor sign with her fingers.*)

Me: What's going on?

Mother: Oh nothing. When we found out it was a bead in the ear, my mom got mad and cut out all the other beads from her hair. She's angry at the stylist because we only got this done last week, so she wants me to call her.

(*Kid pipes up.*)

Kid: Grandma's going to burn it to the ground!

345

Me: What?

Mom, *to kid, annoyed*: I told you, you have to stop saying that! (*To me*) Sorry, my mom was just really upset with the stylist.

Me: Sure, I understand, it's her granddaughter's hair. Well, we'll get this taken care of pretty quickly once they have a room for us.

Mom: Thank you.

Ear foreign body part 3—after the procedure

Finishing up taking out a bead from the kid's ear. Circulator has put the bead in a specimen container.

Circulator: What do you want to do with this? Take it out to show mom? Or send it to Pathology?

Me: Nah, she knows what it is. I mean, I'd love to keep it. Maybe start a little collection. But they don't let you do that anymore. I think I have to send it to Pathology. You know, there was a laryngologist in Philadelphia, Chevalier Jackson, in the early 1900s who kept everything he ever took out.

Circulator: Really?

Me: Yeah, never gave anything back. Even kept a quarter that a kid had aspirated, even though the father beat the kid up for losing the money. He ended up giving the kid fifty cents but kept the quarter.

Circulator: At least the kid doubled his investment.

Me: Gotta be easier ways to make fifty cents than nearly dying.

Circulator: Yeah. Anyway, what should I write on the pathology slip? Bead?

Me: Nah, just write "foreign body." Let them draw their own conclusions. If you want, you can send it in formalin.

Circulator: What, really?

Me: Or we could call the on-call pathologist, maybe get a frozen section. Make sure we really got it all out.

Circulator, *laughing*: Oh, you're joking! I was confused. None of the other ENTs seem to joke around. They're so serious and always in a rush. In fact, most of them would be halfway home right now.

Me: I mean, would I rather be at home playing with my cat and watching TV? Sure. But I'm here, might as well make the most of it. Plus this was a pretty simple thing to do. The kid did great, and the ear looks fine. It all worked out in the end, so might as well add some levity to the situation. It does kinda suck to be stuck in a hospital on a Saturday evening, but there's no point in being surly about it.

Circulator: Well, we appreciate that.

Me: You're welcome.

(THE END.)

Finishing up cauterizing a patient's nose for epistaxis. Walk out of room.

Medical assistant: How did everything go?

Me: Went OK. She had a pretty obvious bleeder along the septum that I cauterized.

MA: Oh good, so nothing like Mr. Sm—

(*I immediately interrupt MA, as she's about to mention the name of a patient who had come to the office for nosebleeds, had a heart attack in the office, required two trips to the OR to control his bleeding as well as two embolizations, and about four further in-office cauterizations.*)

Me: NOPE, DON'T SAY IT.

MA, *starts laughing*: OK, I won't.

Me: I don't ever want to hear that man's name again. Because the universe is always listening, and if we say his name, he's gonna come back.

MA: So you're superstitious?

Me: Definitely! Every surgeon is. You treat his name like You Know Who from Harry Potter. We do not speak of him! We do not speak his name. I don't even want to know if he dies because even then, he'll somehow come back to haunt us with nosebleeds.

MA: OK, got it.

Finishing up seeing a patient and typing the plan in my note

Patient, *watching me type*: Goddamn!

Me: What? What's going on?

Patient: Where did you learn to type?

Me: Oh, I've been typing pretty much my entire life. I learned to type in elementary school.

Patient: But you're so fast!

Me: Yeah, it comes with practice. I do also play the piano.

Patient: It's a good skill to have.

Me: Definitely. But to be honest, in this job, I pretty much type the same fifty words all day. When it's such a small set, you get superquick at typing them.

Patient: Oh.

Me: But thank you. I am proud of my typing ability.

Patient: You're welcome!

Seeing a Patient for "Just Wanted to Make Sure Everything is OK"

Me: So what brings you into the ear, nose, and throat office today?

Patient: I've been making the rounds.

Me: OK, what does that mean?

Patient: I just turned seventy and decided it was a good time to start seeing doctors about my problems. I want to be healthy. So I've seen a cardiologist for my heart, a pulmonologist for my lungs, a nephrologist for my kidneys, and orthopedist for my joints. Everybody says I'm in pretty good shape!

Me: I get the picture. But what brings you to me today?

Patient: I smoke, and my voice has been raspy for twenty-five years. I want to make sure I don't have cancer.

(*Other than smoking, patient doesn't have anything else on history or head/neck exam to suggest cancer. Scope the patient to find she has benign vocal cord swelling.*)

Me: OK, you have what's called Reinke's edema, fancy name for swelling of the vocal cords because of smoking. Everything else looks OK, no masses or lesions or anything else. This is probably the most benign thing that can happen to you from smoking. You should really quit.

(*Patient leans in close to me.*)

Patient: So I'm a very nature-oriented person. I didn't see a doctor for seventy years! I'm not really into pumping my body full of drugs and chemicals. I'm really into holistic healing. Is there anything holistic I can do?

Me: So you don't like drugs and chemicals, but you smoke cigarettes?

Patient: That's natural! Tobacco comes from the ground.

Me: OK, so the most holistic thing you can do is to quit smoking.

Patient: That's it?

Me: Yeah, not just for your voice but for everything!

Seeing a patient for nasal issues

Me: OK, I need to look in the back of the nose with a scope to make sure there are no polyps or masses that might be leading to your sinus problems. I'm going to give you some spray in your nose to numb it and decongest it to make the scope pass a bit easier.

(*Spray up the patient's nose and look at both sides. Takes about thirty seconds or so.*)

Me: OK, we're done.

Patient, *looks at scope*: Oh my god!

Me: I know, I'm sorry, it can be pretty uncomfortable.

Patient: No, it's not that. Can I have a tissue?

Me: Sure, to blow your nose, of course.

(*Grab a tissue and hand it to her.*)

Patient: No, it's not to blow my nose.

(*Patient grabs the scope and wipes it with the tissue.*)

Me: Um, what are you doing?

Patient: My nose is so gross! I don't want you to look at that snot.

Me: It's OK! I've seen much grosser things than your nose.

Patient, *still frantically wiping scope*: I'm so embarrassed.

Me: Don't worry, it's fine! Your nose is just congested, no polyps or masses. Likely just allergies. And please stop trying to clean my scope, you'll end up breaking it. We disinfect it in between every patient. It's not your job to clean my scope!

Patient, *stops and looks at me*: Really?

Me: Really. Plus I don't want you to break it.

(*Patient looks mortified.*)

Me: I mean, you haven't broken it yet, but if you do, I have to charge you $4,000 to replace it. You don't want that.

Patient: Definitely not!

TALES FROM CALL: RECEIVE THE FOLLOWING PAGE

Patient: John Smith

Location: Medical ICU

Message: Patient expired at 12:25 PM.

(*I have never seen this patient before in my life. Call ICU.*)

Me: Hi, this is Dr. Patel with ENT . . .

Secretary: Hold on. (*Yells over shoulder to nurse and then gets back on the phone to me.*) We wanted to let you know that Mr. Smith just died.

Me: Yeah, but I've never seen this patient before. Why am I being called?

Secretary: It's hospital policy. We are required to call every consulting service on a patient if that patient passes away.

(*Hear her flipping through the chart.*)

Secretary: It looks like someone from your practice saw him two weeks ago. That's why you're being called.

Me: You have to call every consultant who has ever seen the patient when they die in the hospital?

Secretary: Yeah, it's a new policy.

Me: That sounds like an incredible waste of time.

Secretary: Yeah, I've had to page eleven doctors for this patient alone!

Me: Yikes, good luck with that. I'll talk to you later.

Secretary: Thanks.

Seeing a patient for "ear pain"

Me: So what brings you in here today?

Patient: My ears have been bothering me for the past three weeks, and I haven't been getting sleep, but I have a three-year-old at home who had the flu two weeks ago, and I also have a newborn who is breastfeeding but was also colicky, and I haven't been sleeping. I keep clenching my jaws together, and the sides of my head hurt. The back of my neck is bothering me. My shoulders are constantly hurting, but that might be because I'm always carrying around both my kids. But also I'm a secretary working full time, and I haven't been sleeping well at all because I have to keep getting up in the middle of the night because my newborn is crying, and my husband keeps saying it's my turn, but I don't think he's helping out too much. But then again he did get up once last night, but then the next time, he told me it was my turn, and I was like, really? It always feels like it's my turn, and I told him I just need some sleep or a break or something because this past weekend, one day, I was actually able to get some sleep for about four to five hours, and my neck and shoulders and back felt better, and my ears were bothering me less, so I was thinking it might all be related to lack of sleep. But I'm not really a doctor, and it could be some sort of brain tumor, and if I die of a brain tumor, I don't know if my husband would be able to take care of these two kids because it doesn't even seem like he can get up in the middle of the night to take care of one kid, let alone two.

(*Long pause.*)

Me, *mostly serious but somewhat facetiously*: How's the stress level?

Patient: It's up there.

Me: So I'm going to take a look at you and make sure there's nothing dangerous going on. But . . . I don't think you have a brain tumor, and I think a lot your symptoms can be explained by lack of sleep and stress.

Patient: Oh definitely. Actually, it feels good to say it all that out loud.

Me: Sometimes that's what you need. A good rant. I can't say that I know what you're going through raising two young kids and working full time, but I think it shows that you're a strong person for trying to accomplish all that.

Patient: Really?

Me: Yeah, keep it in perspective. What you're doing would make anybody lose sleep and be stressed out.

Patient, *laughs*: Well, maybe except my husband.

Me, *hold up my hands*: No comment. This is only an ENT office. All right, let me take a look at your ears.

Finishing up suctioning out a lady's nose after removing packing for epistaxis

Patient: I noticed that you're left-handed.

Me: Yup.

Patient: Wow, so you must have all sorts of left-handed instruments like when you operate!

Me: Nope.

Patient: Really? Why not?

(*Consider it for a moment.*)

Me: I'm not that rich.

Patient, *laughing*: What? Really?

Me: Well, I could go out and buy a whole set of left-handed surgical instruments, but they're very expensive.

Patient: I would have thought they would have given you those things in training.

Me: Are you kidding? They don't do stuff like that for the residents.

Patient: So what did you do?

Me: I figured out how to operate left-handed with the tools they gave me.

Patient: Well, couldn't you have just learned to do it right-handed?

Me: Technically, yes, but it was easier to figure out how to do it left-handed. Sometimes I was forced to do things right-handed, but on the whole, I operated left-handed. Honestly, I think it made me a better surgeon trying to figure out how to do things my way. I'm used to it. Everything in this world is made for you right-handed people anyway, so I've been figuring stuff out like this all my life. Like scissors and screwdrivers and whatnot.

Patient: And the people who trained you? They were OK with that?

Me: Nope, drove them crazy. But whatever. Anyway, your nose looks fine.

Patient: Thank you! And thanks for explaining about the left-handed thing.

Me: You're welcome.

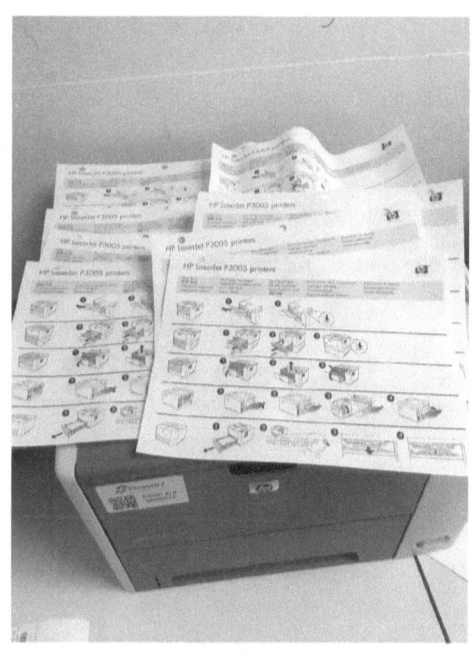

FINISHED UP SEEING A CONSULT IN THE HOSPITAL OVER THE WEEKEND. TRYING TO PRINT THE CONSULT NOTE AND PATIENT FACE SHEET OUT SO I CAN SUBMIT IT FOR BILLING. COMPUTER POPS UP WITH PRINTER ERROR.

Me, *out loud but to myself*: Hm, printer's not working.

Unit secretary: Yeah, it's been acting up all day. Nothing is printing. We called IT, but they're not coming up until Monday.

(*Look at printer, which says "Printer jam—open top cover and back cover and replace."*)

Me: Did anyone up here try to fix it?

Secretary: Well, a bunch of people opened the thing up and then hit the keys, but it still says the thing is broken.

Me: Oh, so you didn't find a paper jam?

Secretary: Apparently not.

(*Open up the top and back covers; find two jammed pieces of paper and remove them.*)

Me: Hm, I think I've isolated the problem.

(*Printer starts printing out test sheets presumably from everyone who hit the large checkmark button.*)

Secretary: Oh wow, you fixed it!

Me: Looks like it. Hey, let's see how many test pages it prints out.

(*Prints out thirteen test pages, with me calling out, "And here's another one!" in between each. Nursing staff is giving me a weird look.*)

Me, *after it finally stops*: OK, should be good to go.

Secretary: Thank you!

Me: You're welcome. Now do you suppose I can bill for that? Disimpaction of printer? 'Cause honestly, what I just did was more satisfying than the garbage consult I just saw. You can just pay me out of pocket too, that's fine.

Secretary: No way.

Me: Ah, well, it was worth a shot. Have a good day.

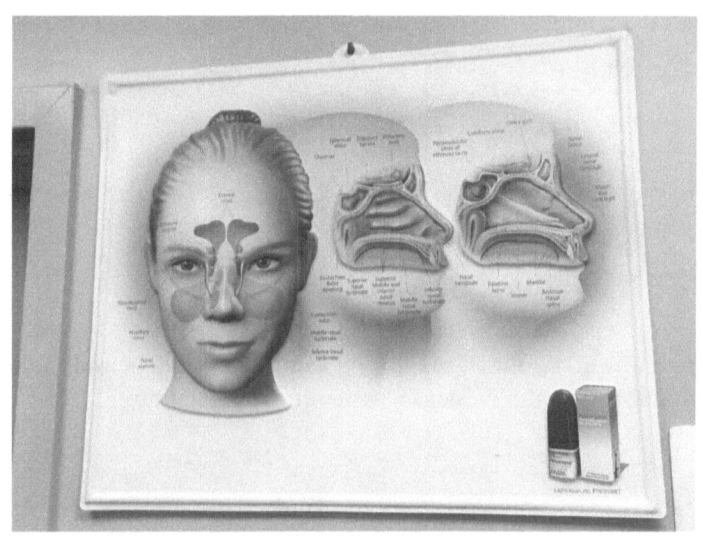

Examining patient's ears; he's looking up at this thing on my wall (see picture).

Patient: Huh.

Me: What's going on?

Patient: That lady in that thing up there for the nose anatomy. She looks like Tonya Harding.

Me, *look at it*: Maybe.

Patient: You're just saying that. You probably have no idea whom I'm talking about. You're too young to know who Tonya Harding is.

Me: I assume you mean Tonya Harding, the ice skater who schemed up a plan with her husband, Jeff Gillooly, to injure Nancy Kerrigan to keep her out of the 1994 Lillehammer Winter Olympics. Unless you mean some other Tonya Harding.

Patient, *startled*: Oh no, that's the one.

Me: They did a parody of it on *Seinfeld*. The episode starred Bette Midler. It was awesome.

Patient: You know what *Seinfeld* is?

Me: Listen, why don't you let me finish examining you first, and then we can chat about what I do and do not know about popular culture?

WAITING TO SEE PATIENTS; CLINIC AIDE COMES IN FLUSTERED.

Aide: I just want to forewarn you about this next patient.

Me: What's up?

Aide: She's here for hearing loss, and it's like pulling teeth to get information or anything. It's just so frustrating.

Me: Why is that?

Aide: She just wants hearing aids and is uninterested in telling me anything else! Apparently, she's had hearing loss since birth, but she just answers in these one-word responses when I'm asking questions. And she didn't come with any information, no previous hearing tests. She's probably never been to see a doctor before.

Me: Well, maybe not.

Aide: And this is going to sound really judgmental, but she's got dreadlocks, and the guy that's with her has tattoos all over his arms.

Me, *perplexed*: That does sound judgmental. What has that got to do with anything?

Aide: I don't know, you just get the sense that they're clueless. I mean, I'm just trying to help them, but they're making it really difficult.

Me: Well, maybe they are clueless, but that might not be their fault. Maybe this lady has had issues with access to care and couldn't see a primary care doctor let alone a specialist. Or maybe nobody ever tried to really explain what was going on with the hearing loss, so she didn't know to come with any previous records. Who knows? Also, lots of people have dreadlocks and tattoos. That doesn't have anything to do with why they're here.

Aide, *considers for a moment*: Yeah, I guess that could be true. Huh, now you're making me feel bad about this.

Me: Well, maybe you should feel bad a little bit. But let's at least try to educate this lady about her problem. Give her the tools to make an informed decision. It might be as simple as a hearing aid, but who knows? Maybe they need some sort of surgery. We have to try. That's all we can do.

Aide: All right, that's fair.

Finishing up for the day; medical assistant walks in.

MA: Just to let you know, I added five earwax removal patients for you tomorrow. An entire family. They're leaving on vacation this weekend and want their ears cleaned before they leave.

Me: Very funny. That's a great joke. Who gets their ears cleaned before a vacation?

MA: I'm not joking.

Me: Wait, what?

(*Look at schedule, and there are five appointments in a row, the Smith family (mom and four kids), whom I've seen before.*)

Me: Wow, OK. Five cerumen patients right in a row. Are you trying to make my head explode?

MA: I'm sorry.

Me: I'm only kidding. At least it's not dizziness. I would have just quit if that were the case. And at least I've seen them all before. Actually, it's kind of funny.

MA: Why?

Me: So this family consists of a set of identical triplets and their elder brother. I didn't know they were triplets at the time because their mother brought them in one at a time over the course of three days. Then she brought the elder brother in on the fourth day, and he looks exactly like the triplets too. I felt like I was in the Twilight Zone or something or one of the nine circles of hell, just constantly cleaning the same set of ears over and over again. So maybe it's better I get it all over in one shot.

MA: Maybe. We'll see.

A Story of Two Cerumen Patients

Patient 1: young woman in the Coast Guard.

Patient: I hate having my ears cleaned. It's the worst pain in the world. It's worse than giving childbirth.

Me: Really? That bad, huh? Well, I'm going to at least try, but if it's too painful, we'll stop, I'll give you a break, and we'll try again. If you're absolutely unable to tolerate it altogether, we'll stop.

(*Pick up suction and begin cleaning ears.*)

Patient, *after approximately ten seconds*: Oh my god, oh my god, oh my god, YOU HAVE TO STOP!

Me, *stopping*: Is it hurting?

Patient: No, I'm just freaking out! Give me a second!

(*Patient puts her head between her knees and breathes deeply for thirty seconds and then lets me try again. We repeat this cycle for a good fifteen minutes until her ears are clean.*)

Patient: I'm sorry, I'm such a baby. I must be the worst patient you have.

Me: Not the worst. Some people try to take swings at me. Certainly not the best either, but that's OK.

Patient 2: two year-old who had ear tubes placed eight months ago, coming in for follow up. Both ears packed with wax.

Me, *to mom*: Well, I'm going to have to clean out her ears to figure out what's going on with those tubes. I'll try my best, but kiddos usually squirm around too much for me to do anything. We might just have to put her on some drops.

Mom: She'll be OK. Let me just put something on my phone to watch.

Me, *skeptical*: OK.

(*Mom opens an app, which starts singing.*)

"Five little monkeys jumping on the bed.

One fell off and bumped his head.

Mama called the doctor,

And the doctor said,

No more monkeys jumping on the bed . . ."

And so on and so forth.

(*Kid doesn't move once, even when I use forceps to remove an extruded tube sitting on the eardrum.*)

Me, *to mom*: She did amazing! That was really unexpected.

Mom: Thanks!

Me: No, you really don't understand. She was literally one of the best patients I've had, including adults. You have no idea how some people carry on about getting their ears cleaned, and here's a two-year old that was perfect. By the way, what app was that?

Mom: Well, thank you! That was just some nursery rhyme app.

Me: Hm, maybe I should have that ready to go for some of these adult patients. Or better yet, a video of me cleaning your daughter's ears to show those adults so they won't complain as much.

Mom, *laughs*: Well, maybe next time.

SEEING A PATIENT FOR TINNITUS

Me: So it says here that you have ringing in your ears. How long has that been going on for?

Patient: About three weeks or so.

Me: Anything that happened three weeks ago that you think may have set it off?

Patient: I was in Florida, and I was reading an article in a magazine about ringing in the ears, and all of a sudden, I noticed that I had that.

(*Long silence.*)

Me: You read an article about tinnitus and developed tinnitus?

Patient: Yeah, then I read about tinnitus on the Internet and saw that it can be caused by a brain tumor or MS, so I want to make sure I don't have those. Maybe I need an MRI or a spinal tap or something.

Me: OK.

(*Finish up my history and examine patient; everything is extremely benign, and he has a mild high-frequency hearing loss symmetrically.*)

Me: OK, I'm going to ask you a question.

Patient: OK . . .

Me: Don't think about elephants. What's the first thing you think about?

Patient: Elephants.

Me: That's probably what's going on here. The tinnitus has likely been going on for a long time, and now that you're thinking about it, you're hearing it. I don't think you have MS or a brain tumor, and I think it's probably overkill to go ordering MRIs or other tests. I think you just need to focus on identifying those times when you're hearing the tinnitus and use something like a white noise machine or radio tuned to soft static to distract your brain.

Patient: Really?

Me: Really. Obviously, if anything changes, come back, and we'll reevaluate things. By the way, have you ever seen the movie *Inception*?

Patient: No.

Me: You should watch it. It might give you some perspective on what's going on.

Patient: Oh OK. Is it a documentary?

Me: Not really. But it's a good movie.

SEEING A PATIENT FOR A COLD GOING ON FOR TWO DAYS

Me: So no issues with your sinuses at all? No allergies or recurrent infections?

Patient: No, nothing like that.

Me: So nasal congestion and a drip with a mild cough for two days?

Patient: Yeah.

Me: No fevers or chills?

Patient: No way.

Me: Out of curiosity, why did you come to see me about this? Do you want surgery?

Patient: Oh god, no!

Me: Because usually, when someone comes to an ENT for sinus issues, they're coming to consider surgery.

Patient: No, I wasn't able to get an appointment with my primary doctor for three whole days after this started, and I was afraid the symptoms would go away before I got a chance to see her. Plus you had an opening according to your website, so I figured I'd see you.

Me: OK . . .

Patient: Yeah, I'm pretty healthy overall. No major medical issues. I take a lot of vitamins—vitamin A, B6, B12, a lot of vitamin C because you know, they all say that vitamin C is really good for you. I don't like taking medications, but I like taking vitamins. I take zinc too and sometimes calcium and vitamin D, you know, for bone health. You know what I do when I start to get a cold though?

(*To be honest, I'm only half listening to the patient at this point.*)

Me: Hm, what's that?

Patient: Well, I told you about the vitamin C. So I eat a grapefruit every morning. Grapefruit is very good for you. Do you eat grapefruit?

Me: Not on a regular basis, no.

Patient: Well, if I can offer you some medical advice, start eating one every day. Anyway, when I start to get a cold, I start eating ANOTHER grapefruit at lunch, and it takes care of it.

Me: Great.

Patient: But this cold seems to be lingering.

Me: After two days?

Patient: Well, I was thinking, and I want to run this by you. I want to start eating another grapefruit at dinnertime. Do you think that's OK?

Me: So you want to bump up the grapefruit dose from twice daily to three times daily?

Patient: Yes, is that all right?

Me: I think that's absolutely fine. I think you're going to be OK. Just keep going with the supportive care things, nasal saline, salt water gargles, steam inhalation. And if it continues to be an issue, please see your primary care doctor.

Patient: And the grapefruit, right?

Me: Sure.

Seeing a ninety-year-old man for imbalance/dizziness

Me: I don't think this is necessarily related to your inner ear. You seem to have some significant mobility issues though.

Patient: Yeah, my hips have been bothering me for years. They're really stiff, and I always have to be close to a wall to hang on because I feel unsteady. I'm ninety years old though. I don't want one of those surgeries or anything.

Me: I'm not saying you need to have surgery, but have you considered a cane or a walker?

Patient: That will make me look old!

Me: Fair enough. You are ninety years old, though, so getting up there. And if you need it, you need it. Worse thing that can happen here is you fall over and really injure yourself.

Patient: I hear what you're saying. You know, it's nice talking to you.

Me: Thank you. It's nice talking to you too!

Patient: You know, that's a real problem. I used to just sit and talk with my general doctor but he just recently retired! It was nice.

Me: That does sound nice.

Patient: You know what the other problem is?

Me: What's that?

Patient: My wife of seventy years died a few months ago. She used to do everything for me. It's been so tough without her. She used to do a lot.

Me: I'm very sorry to hear that.

Patient, *tearing up*: I can't think of her without crying. You know what I do now? You're going to think I'm crazy.

Me: Well, not yet.

Patient: Every night, I take her picture and sit it next to me, and we watch TV together. And I talk to her. I know she's gone, but I still like talking to her. I really miss her.

Me: That's not crazy at all. My mother died about three years ago, and I still really miss her.

Patient: You and me, we're peas in a pod, huh?

Me: Something like that. We're all done for today, but if you want to come back to talk, you're more than welcome.

Patient: You're very nice to say that, but I'll go bother someone else.

Me: Fair enough.

(*Patient leaves. MA walks in.*)

MA: You made that nice man cry? Why?

Me: Eh, he was lonely and wanted someone to talk to.

MA: You didn't torture him?

Me: Not at all, I swear!

Cleaning out an eighty-year-old lady's ears

Patient, *yelling because she's very hard of hearing*: I HOPE YOU'RE READY!

Me: For wax? Always.

Patient: I HAVE VERY NARROW EAR CANALS! I'M A MESS!

Me: Well, let me clean out your ears so your hearing aids have a chance to work.

Patient: THAT WOULD MAKE ME A HAPPY MESS!

Me: Great.

(*Clean out patient's ears; ear canals are narrow but normal, and everything else looks OK.*)

Me: OK, you're all cleaned out.

Patient: LET ME SEE THE WAX!

Me: Um, OK.

(*Show her the wax.*)

Patient: OH MY GOD, THERE'S SO MUCH!

Me: I wouldn't say it's a lot but enough to cause you some problems.

Patient: LISTEN, SHOULD I HAVE IT TESTED?

Me: Have what tested? Your wax? Test it for what?

Patient: I DON'T KNOW! YOU'RE THE DOCTOR! WAX ISN'T NORMAL!

Me: I assure you, wax is normal. And we don't test it for anything.

Patient: OH OK. SO I'LL MAKE AN APPOINTMENT TO COME BACK NEXT WEEK FOR THE SAME THING?

Me: Next week? That's way too soon.

Patient: BUT MY EARS NEED CLEANING ON A REGULAR BASIS!

Me: OK, why don't you just come back when it's bothering you? Let's say six months.

Patient: THAT'S WAY TOO LONG!

Me: OK, just make an appointment for whenever you'd like, and I'll take a look in your ears.

Patient: OK!

(Another life saved.)

Finishing up a parathyroidectomy with a surgical resident

Resident: Any special orders?

Me: Not really. He can go to a floor bed. Just get a calcium level this evening and tomorrow morning.

Resident: OK.

(*Later in the day, I log into the medical record system and find that my patient is in the ICU. Call the resident in a mild amount of panic.*)

Me: Hey, what happened? Why is my patient in the ICU?

Resident: Oh, there's no more surgical floor beds available, so we had to put him in the ICU.

Me: Jesus, they must love that admission.

(*Go to ICU and see patient, who's doing great, and then go to talk to the nurse.*)

ICU Nurse: Yeah, he's doing fine.

Me: So this is probably your easiest admission ever, right?

Nurse: Oh definitely. A walking, talking patient who's voiding on his own? I'll take one of those any day.

Me: Great.

Seeing a young lady for ear issues

Me: What brings you in here today?

Patient: My primary care doctor looked in my ears and said I really needed to see an ENT.

Me: Hm, OK.

Patient: Yeah, so I use bobby pins to scratch my ears. I'm trying to break the habit, but it feels so good. Do you know what I mean?

Me: Not me personally, but I know quite a few people that use Q-tips for that exact reason.

Patient: Also, my earwax smells really bad, like for a while now. Do you know how earwax can sometimes really smell bad?

Me: I usually don't make it a habit of smelling earwax.

Patient: Well, this is where we are.

Me: Fair enough, you feel like your earwax has started smelling bad. I'll take a look and see what's going on.

(*Look in ears, see a chronic fungal infection on both sides, and it does smell terrible.*)

Patient: So what's going on?

Me: You have what looks like a chronic fungal infection in both ears.

Patient: That's so gross!

Discontinue Leeches!!
And Other Stories from an ENT's Training

Me: It is gross. But I'm going to put you on some drops, and we're going to try to get this under control. And you have to stop using the bobby pins to scratch your ears!

Patient: I know, I'm trying. I read somewhere it takes thirty days to stop a habit, and I'm a week off bobby pins.

Me: That's great!

Patient: Yeah, I feel like I deserve a one-week token.

Me: Like Bobby Pins Anonymous? I'm not sure that exists.

Finishing up doing a flexible nasal endoscopy

Patient: Ugh, I'm so sorry if was a bad patient.

Me: Nah, you did fine!

Patient: I don't know why I hate that so much.

Me: Well, you hate it because it feels weird. It's not normal to have something shoved up your nose. Noses don't like it.

Patient: Yeah, I guess you're right.

Me: Actually, I've only had one person say afterward he really liked the experience.

Patient: Really?

Me: Yeah, but he was a bit weird. Anyway, I'm not offended if you hate having a scope done.

Patient: Oh OK.

TALKING WITH A FRIEND WHO IS A CARDIOLOGIST

Cardiologist: I'm supposed to lead a suturing class for students. I last did that ten years ago. Should I get chicken?

Me: Or pig feet.

Cardiologist: Where do you get those?

Me: Supermarket should have them depending on where you go. Otherwise, chicken is fine. Out of curiosity, do you do a lot of suturing?

Cardiologist: No. Just pacemaker pockets.

Me: Nice.

Cardiologist: You would probably laugh if you saw me.

Me: Probably. Call a surgical consult.

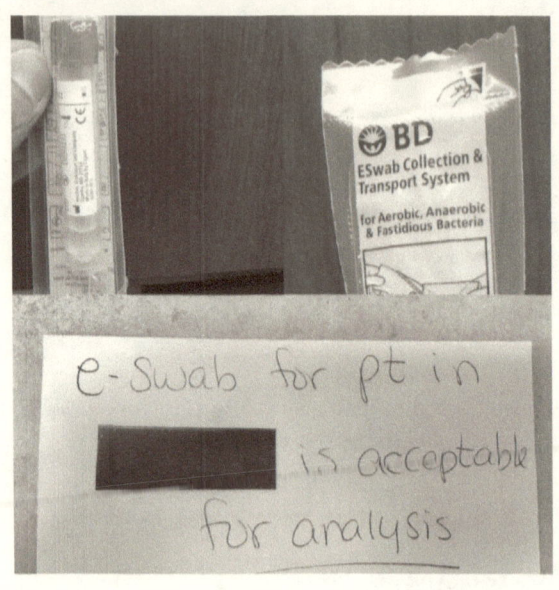

CALLED FOR PAROTITIS (INFECTION OF SALIVARY GLAND) IN A DEMENTED COMBATIVE DEHYDRATED LADY. SEE PUS COMING FROM THE GLAND DUCT IN THE MOUTH. AS PHYSICIANS WE'RE TAUGHT, IF YOU SEE PUS, IT SHOULD BE CULTURED (ESPECIALLY IF IT HAS NOT BEEN CULTURED BEFORE). I ASK THE NURSE TO GET ME A CULTURE SWAB.

Nurse, *hands me two of the pictured culture swab*: This is all we have on the floor.

Me: Hm... I'm used to the red-top swab. But this does say for aerobic, anaerobic, and fastidious bacterial culture. Looks like it will work. Thanks!

Discontinue Leeches!!
And Other Stories from an ENT's Training

(Because patient is demented and combative, nurse has to hold down her arms while I depress the tongue and take the culture. I sit down to write up the consult and get a call from the lab.)

Lab secretary: Hi, Dr. Patel, we can't accept this culture swab. It was collected incorrectly. The lab tech says it needs to be in the red-top tube.

Me: Really? Even though the swab I used is for bacterial culture?

Secretary: Um, that's what she says. Let me put you on with her.

(Transfers me to lab tech.)

Lab tech: We only use those blue-top tubes for influenza, not bacterial culture.

Me: OK, let me read this off to you. It says, "ESwab collection and transport system for aerobic, anaerobic, and fastidious bacteria." Doesn't say anything about flu. Maybe you're thinking of another blue-top tube?

Lab tech: No, I know the one you're talking about. We use them for flu culture only.

Me: You're using a bacterial swab for a viral culture? Is that what you said? Because again, it says nothing on here about flu or viral culture.

Lab tech: To be honest, we send these things out to another hospital for analysis, and there's no way they'll accept the blue-top tube. Let me connect you to my boss so she can explain that to you.

(Transfers me to lab boss, and I explain situation.)

Lab boss: We really only accept the red-top tubes for bacterial culture. The blue-top tubes are used for nasal swabs only. The nose has different bacteria than other parts of the—

Me, *very calmly*: So I'm going to cut you off here. I'm an ear, nose, and throat doctor, and I know a fair amount about the nose. There's nothing on this culture swab that says it needs to be used exclusively in the nose, only that it's for aerobic, anaerobic, and fastidious bacteria. Also, your tech just told me you use these tubes for viral culture, and I admit I'm not the smartest person in the world, but it doesn't seem like you should be using bacterial culture swabs for viral culture. If you only want blue-top tubes used for nasal culture, that's fine, but you should label them that way, even though that's ridiculous. It seems to me like you guys have no idea what's going on up here or what tubes are used for what reasons, which is odd for a hospital lab. And last, I had to torture this lady to get this culture swab. If you'd like me to go torture this lady again to get a red-top culture swab, I'll go do it.

Lab boss: Well, I don't want you to torture her, that's not why she's here. Let me call the other hospital to see if it's acceptable medium for transport. You know, you're the first doctor that's run into this issue.

Me: Seems unlikely. But you guys need to figure out how to fix this.

(*Give the lady my office number, and when I get to the office, they hand me the pictured note.*)

(To comment: In medicine, we're asked to put up with a lot of ridiculousness. Most of the time we're happy to go along with it in the name of patient care. To get upset at every silly thing that happens in a hospital would be paralyzing. However, every now and again, you do have to call out blatant bullshit when you see it. And it's always fun to counteract stupidity with cool logic explained to the offending party in a simple way.)

Walk into a room for cerumen removal in a ninety-six-year-old lady with hearing aids. She's there with her son and a health-care aide.

Me: Hi, my name is Dr. Patel.

Patient: OH, LOOK AT HIM! HE'S A YOUNG ONE!

Me: Well, I guess that's true.

Patient: BUT THEN, EVERYONE IS YOUNG TO ME! I'M PUSHING ONE HUNDRED!

Me: That's great!

Patient, *looking around*: I HOPE YOU'RE NOT CLAUSTROPHOBIC!

Me: What, because of the size of the room? Nah, I'm not claustrophobic. But you're right, it is a small room.

Patient, *points at my fleece*: AREN'T YOU HOT? IT'S SO WARM OUTSIDE!

Me: Well, it would only be an issue if they let me have my office hours outside. They keep it unbelievably cold in here. I know I'm ludicrously attired.

Patient: YOU GOT THAT RIGHT!

Me: Very good. Let's clean out those ears, shall we?

(*Clean out the wax from both sides.*)

Patient: SOUND'S LIKE YOU WERE CLEANING A JUNKYARD OUT OF THERE!

Me: Not the worst I've ever seen.

Patient: YOU'RE JUST SAYING THAT! I KNOW MY EARS!

Me: That's true. After ninety-six years with them, you probably do. Well, you're good to go.

I FEEL LIKE THIS MIGHT BE A REPEATING THEME OR HAVE POSTED A STORY LIKE IT BEFORE BUT . . . GET CALLED FOR "EAR PAIN" IN-PATIENT CONSULT AT 3:00 PM.

Nurse: This patient has left ear pain.

Me: OK, what is the patient admitted there for?

Nurse: For ear pain.

Me: What, really? How long have they been there for? They were admitted today?

Nurse: Oh no. The patient has been here for two days.

Me: And you're calling now? I don't understand. Has an ENT seen this patient before?

Nurse: No. This is the first time we're calling you.

Me: So a patient that has had such bad ear pain that they got admitted to the hospital two days ago hasn't been seen by an ENT. Something's not adding up. What does the admitting doctor say?

(*Hear nurse shuffling through the chart.*)

Nurse: I'm not sure.

Me: OK . . . Did someone look in the ear?

Nurse: No.

Me: So you're telling me that a patient was admitted to the hospital for ear pain, no one looked in the ear, and they've been there for two days? That's what you're saying?

Nurse: Yes.

Me: Because that sounds really stupid.

Nurse: Oh wait, here it is. Patient was admitted for cardiac workup and is on telemetry, but he was to be discharged today. He's been complaining of pain in the left ear for six years. He's unhappy with the ENT he saw six years ago and wants another one. We canceled his discharge this morning pending ENT consult.

Me: OK, he's had ear pain for six years, and you've been holding him in the hospital for me to come see him?

Nurse: Yes.

Me: So I'm not going to come and see him. You can discharge him, and he can make an appointment to be seen in the office. Ear pain for six years is the definition of a nonurgent consult. I know you're just doing your job, but for your own edification, if you or a physician is going to call an ENT for an ear consult, you better look in the patient's ears. I don't even care if you know what you're looking at, but you have to do the very basics. I'm not a walking otoscope. That's not what I do.

Nurse: No, I understand.

Me: Great, thanks!

> I was moonlighting on a medical unit, sitting in the Doctor office
>
> Nurse calls the office phone to ask if I have an otoscope
>
> I said "no, why?"
>
> "There's an ent resident here and he forgot his and he seems upset that we don't have one"
>
> "Uh...ill look in this office"
>
> I open one drawer, find some trident gum, of which I take a piece and find very refreshing
>
> Then I walked out to the nurse's desk where the ENT resident was
>
> With a stapler that I found in the office
>
> And I asked "is this what you were looking for?"

   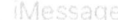

AND FINALLY, I RECEIVE THE ABOVE TEXT MESSAGE FROM A CARDIOLOGIST FRIEND WHILE WAITING ON MY LAST PATIENT OF THE AFTERNOON ONE DAY.

To be honest, that ENT resident deserved what happened.

The world of medicine continues to be absurd.

www.ingramcontent.com/pod-product-compliance
Lightning Source LLC
Chambersburg PA
CBHW020722180526

45163CB00001B/70